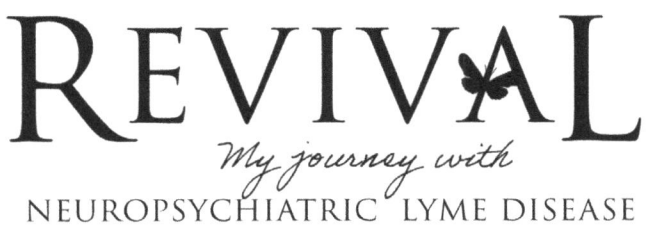

NEUROPSYCHIATRIC LYME DISEASE

KAITLYN OLEINIK

REVIVAL
My Journey with Neuropsychiatric Lyme Disease

by KAITLYN OLEINIK

Copyright ©2025 by Kaitlyn Oleinik

All rights reserved.

This book or part thereof may not be reproduced in any form by any means, electronic or mechanical, including photocopy, recording, or otherwise, or by any information storage and retrieval system, except as may be expressly permitted in writing from the publisher as provided by the United States of America copyright law. Visit www.ChantillyPress.org for permission requests.

Published by

Chantilly Press, Orange County, CA

Cover by Fiona Jayde Media
Interior design by The Deliberate Page

Electronic ISBN: 979-8-9986924-0-6
Paperback ISBN: 979-8-9986924-1-3
Paperback ISBN: 979-8-9986924-9-9
Hardcover ISBN: 979-8-9986924-2-0

Library of Congress Control Number 2025907923

This is a personal history work and is not meant to be taken as medical advice. THIS BOOK DOES NOT PROVIDE MEDICAL ADVICE. The information, including but not limited to, text, graphics, images and other material contained in this book are solely of the opinion of the author and for informational purposes only. No material contained herein is intended to be a substitute for professional medical advice, diagnosis or treatment. ALWAYS SEEK THE ADVICE OF YOUR PHYSICIAN or other qualified health care provider with any questions you may have regarding a medical condition or treatment, and before undertaking a new health care regimen, and never disregard professional medical advice or delay seeking it because of something you have read on the pages in this book. Any resemblance to actual persons, living or dead, including events and locations, is entirely coincidental.

Table of Contents

My Story 1

A Message from Kaitlyn 3

Delusion 7

   1: Reality 9

The POWER of the PAST 13

   2: It All Began with a Little Bug 15

   3: Incessantly Infected 19

   4: The Physical Insult Continues 25

ACTIONS and REACTIONS 29

   5: Possibilities 31

   6: Pretty Sick Dancer 37

   7: Heat 41

   8: "Butterfly" Symptoms 51

   9: Gym Time 55

   10: Brain Fog 59

   11: Back to School 63

   12: Relationships 69

   13: Gaslighting 73

   14: Enter POTS 81

   15: Ski Season and a Cry For Help 83

   16: "It's Just Anxiety?" 89

   17: Not the guy 93

- 18: My Grandma, Uncle, and a Betta Fish 95
- 19: Loss 99
- 20: Fear for My safety 103
- 21: Music and the Influencer Era 105
- 22: Lyme Literacy 111
- 23: Tests, Tests, and More Tests 113
- 24: A New Friend and an LLMD 117
- 25: There's Something Inside of Me 121
- 26: Not the Antidote. 125
- 27: Out of Control. 127
- 28: Back Again. 131

Disorder: The Great Educator 137

- 29: Psychosis 139
- 30: Group Revelation 141
- 31: It's All on the Internet 147
- 32: Heiress Apparent 151
- 33: Weight Peak and Back to School 155
- 34: Mediterranean Diet. 159
- 35: With the Help of GLP-1 Medications 163
- 36: Back to One-der-land 167
- 37: Bachelor's Degree at Last. 171
- 38: Grad School. 173
- 39: The Board of Pharmacy. 179

For Your Information 181

- FYI—Let's Talk About Options 183
- End Statement 207
- References. 209
- About the Author 213

My Story

"The only source of knowledge is experience. You learn a lot by trying things out and seeing what happens"

~ Albert Einstein

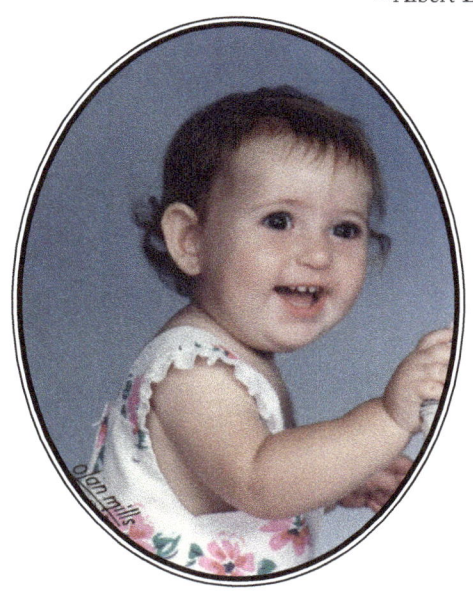

A Message from Kaitlyn

I write this book to break "stigma." This is the story of what happened to me. I have been told "we are only as sick as our secrets" (Alcoholics Anonymous)… so, I am setting mine free with the hopes that they help someone.

When I was young and struggling, I was told to keep those trials secret, and as a result, couldn't have felt more alone. I think the more we talk about our struggles, the more we can also talk about our resilience and the ability to bounce back from terrible things that have happened to us. The title of this book was inspired by a Selena Gomez (who is diagnosed with bipolar disorder) song and era—*Revival*.

Revival is defined as "An improvement in the condition or strength of something."

Not only did I do that, I experienced a rebirth. My entire life as I knew it blew up when I relapsed from late-stage neurological Lyme disease that turned into neuropsychiatric Lyme that triggered a 105 pound inflammation-driven weight gain.

I lost my friends, my mind, and my body as I recognized it. I had to heal from the ground up and heal years of trauma to reclaim life and brain, and not only get back on track, but transform again into the person I knew I was always meant to be. I found purpose again and fought to be the person I wanted to be.

As Selena Gomez says, "This is more than my survival, this is my revival."

Kaitlyn Oleinik

Here is the story of my survival… the path of revival from late-stage neuropsychiatric Lyme disease.

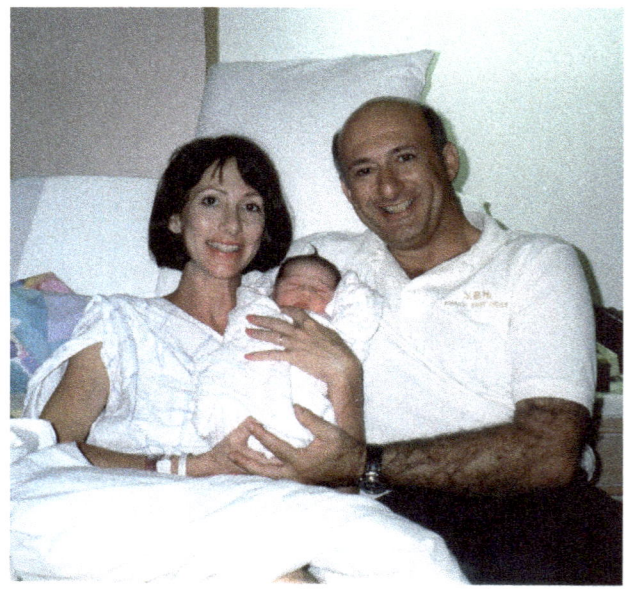

My Birthday

MEDICAL ADVICE DISCLAIMER

DISCLAIMER: THIS BOOK DOES NOT PROVIDE MEDICAL ADVICE. The information, including but not limited to, text, graphics, images and other material contained in this book are solely of the opinion of the author and for informational purposes only. No material contained herein is intended to be a substitute for professional medical advice, diagnosis or treatment. ALWAYS SEEK THE ADVICE OF YOUR PHYSICIAN or other qualified health care provider with any questions you may have regarding a medical condition or treatment, and before undertaking a new health care regimen, and never disregard professional medical advice or delay seeking it because of something you have read on the pages in this book.

I knew this was my death… or my revival.

(Journal entry, 2019)

Delusion

"Am I getting a brain scan?"

The answer came from a young nurse, too occupied with his paperwork to look at me. "No, psych ward," was all he said.

My throat seemed to shrink to the size of a straw and my gut clenched. *What is happening?* No one said anything. No one looked at me. I didn't exist in this place—just a number in the computer with the initials S. O. next to it. Not one person noticed the scrub pants soaked in urine, the ones I wore with my t-shirt with the hole in the back. I'm not even sure how the urine got there, though someone said I'd done it.

"You don't understand," I said to a young girl walking past me with towels in her hands. "It's not my fault. It's the damn tick bite."

She didn't look at me either.

I looked at my wrists, still red from where the handcuffs had been. "It's not my fault," I said to no one, glancing at my leg where the bite had been so many years ago.

"Hey, Kaitlyn," a male voice said. *No one looks at me, so I won't look at you.* "I'm going to take your vitals again."

He is just trying to get you to look at him. The thought raced through my head, along with the voice of my favorite rapper. *He was going to save me. He was supposed to finish his rapping, my favorite song, then pick me up…* "on the freeway." The thought finished itself and I heard my own voice speak. *That male taking my vital signs is trying to get me to say more. Fine. I'll answer.* "Never mind. They just wanted to finish filming the Wizard of Oz with me and I had to walk. You wouldn't know, but that was the first time I could walk without pain. Did you even consider that?"

I could tell I wasn't making sense to him, but everything made perfect sense to me. My inflamed brain wouldn't stop, and neither would my tongue.

No reply as he hit the button to start the blood pressure cuff. It squeezed my bicep and I flinched. "That hurts, though. But my walking didn't. Do you even care?"

No response.

I could tell that he didn't. There was no empathy there. None from the police either who made me sit in those urine-soaked scrubs in the back seat.

"No one cares. But maybe someone cares about my dad. Did anyone check on him?"

He took the cuff from my arm, and I heard scuffling in the room and closed my eyes tighter so I wouldn't look.

"No." The defiance in my voice seemed to help against the nausea that began to climb from my clenched stomach into my throat.

Why didn't anyone care? Why didn't someone just ask me, "Kaitlyn why did you run down the street, barefoot, at night like that? Where were you going when the police picked you up?"

The room was empty again. No one bothered to ask how I was doing or what I was doing. No one cared.

I cleared my throat and whispered. "Because I thought they were going to kill me!"

1:
Reality

That night was one of the worst nights of my life. I had just finished several rounds of stem cell infusions and strong antibiotics. The outcome was a 5150 psych-hold—the result of a delusional event that landed me in the back of a police car and then the Emergency Department's psych room. Perhaps the treatments had been too much for my brain, all at once, but no one addressed that. Again, no one cared, and everyone thought I had gone crazy.

Perhaps so… but the cause was not organic, it was due to a bite that had been treated with too many methodologies, medications, therapies, and such from both western and eastern medicine "expert" approaches. This is called an "integrative" approach to medicine and I believed that the combination of practices would be beneficial. Time proved them all to be wrong, and I suffered because of it. Fortunately, the tides turned and improvement was forthcoming… albeit slowly.

During the time of my delusion, several events took place in my physique, two of which caused tremendous trauma to my already frail psyche: I gained massive weight despite not eating much at all, and then the belief crept in that parasites had invaded my body. The only answer to the second dilemma was to shave the hair from off my skin in hopes that the parasites would abandon their host. So, I took scissors to my scalp and a razor to my eyebrows. The lesions were painful, but not as painful as the delusions.

"She's just fat!"

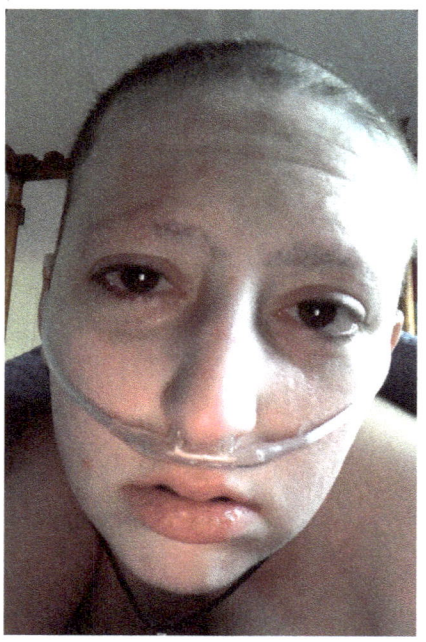

That was the expert doctor's response to the 70 pounds I had suddenly gained. No one spoke of the classic "moon face" I'd donned since starting on steroids, or the insulin resistance that followed it… only that I was fat and should cut down on my food intake while increasing my activity.

The simple fact was that I couldn't walk.

I couldn't walk to the fridge or to the kitchen or to the pantry, and especially not down the street to McDonalds to get food. The assumption that I had been overeating to cause such weight gain was preposterous. Even I knew that to be true. Not all obesity is a result of calories in/calories out. Not all mental illness is genetic or organic. Not all symptoms of illness are easily recognized. But many are very easily dismissed by physicians who want to see what they want to diagnose. There's a saying that speaks volumes to what I experienced:

"To a surgeon, every problem needs a scalpel."

It's called *confirmation bias* in the medical journals, and I was its victim.

This all happened in 2020, and years would pass before I had fully recovered. In truth, my issues were not considered unique, but at that time, they were rare. And the simple fact remains… I have Lyme disease and this is my story.

The POWER of the PAST

> *"Those who cannot remember the past
> are condemned to repeat it."*
>
> ~ George Santayana

2:
It All Began with a Little Bug

The white brush smelled amazing the weekend we took our family trip to the bluff. The little town of Poplar Bluff was rustic and rural, a perfect place for a family to reunite, recreate, and build memories. Doug was notorious for creating great memories with the cousins. This was especially true on the river. Our favorite was to float down Black River on inflated inner tubes.

"Wait!" Doug shouted at me. He was my mom's cousin and someone I trusted.

I had floated only a few yards from him on my inner tube but obviously, he was nervous about something. He quickly paddled over to me and began to inspect my legs that stuck out behind me in the river.

"What?" I replied, wondering what was going on.

"Wait. Stop. Let me see…" he continued and took hold of my leg by the ankle. "There!" he said, picking at something on the back of my thigh. He then wiped it off and splashed water all over my legs. "You had something on your thigh. I think it was a tick."

"Ewww. Gross," was my reply, and no further thought was given to the incident.

Little did I know that single event would change my life forever.

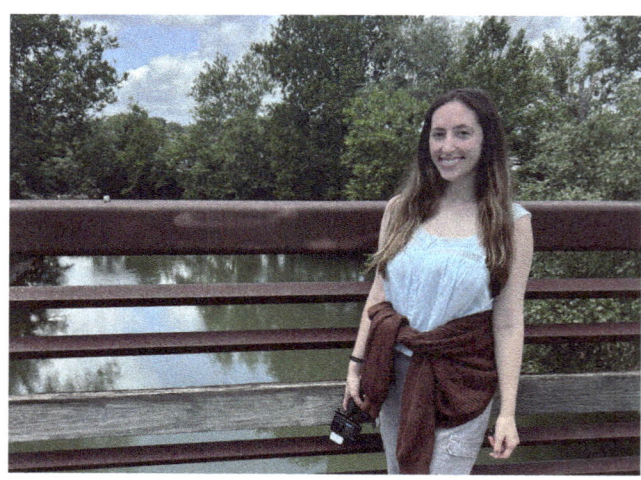

Black River (Revisited)

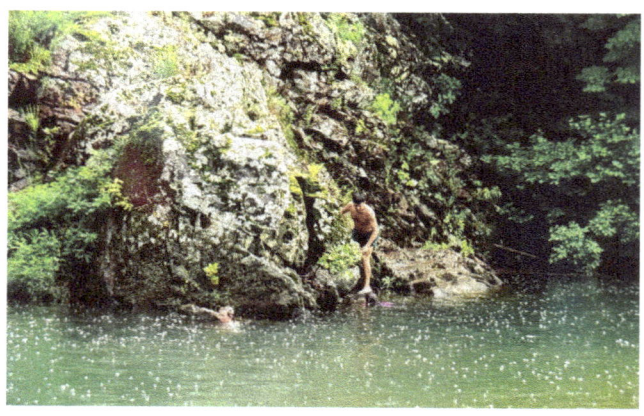

Summer of 2000, the day the tick was found on my leg

2: It All Began with a Little Bug

I'm not 100% certain that the tick on my thigh was the perpetrator of my disease. However, the likelihood is high. Of course, there may have been another (or more) tick on me during that trip, but none was found—only the predator stuck to my thigh.

For those unfamiliar with tick biology, they can be as small as a pinhead and very difficult to see with the naked eye. So, the possibility that I had been bitten at another time is real, but the happenstance that a tick found on my leg, witnessed by someone other than myself, and the resulting illness is rather coincidental.

The timeline of the resulting disease was not coincidental, however. By age ten, I was in full neurological symptomatic illness. Few were ready to admit what was going on and few others had no idea. My childhood was about to be racked with issues most never hear about.

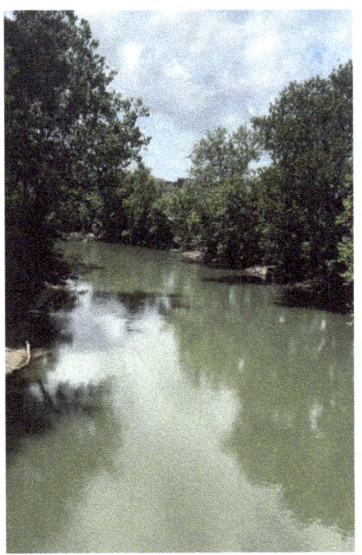 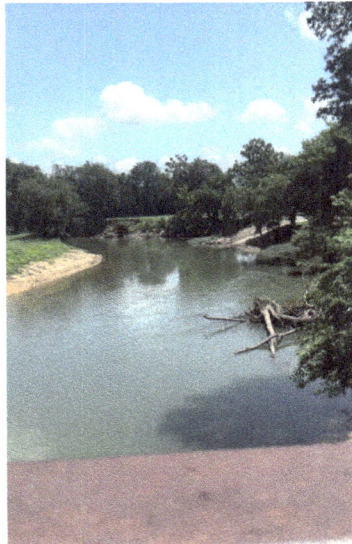

Black River

3:
Incessantly Infected

Every year, from the time of early childhood, I would suffer with a sinus infection. The traditional management for these types of infections was a course of antibiotics. Round after round of medications introduced a steady outbreak of rashes due to the bombardment on my body of these antibiotics, many of which were administered prior to any resolution of the current rash. I'm still unsure whether the antibiotics or my weakened immune system reacted first, but the end result was severe allergy to several of the medications I had been given in those years.

Despite the illnesses and irritating rashes, I led a normal, active life as a child. My parents say my energy level was average for a kid—full of activity, singing, dancing, performing—days filled with school, friends, art, and music. My favorite was dance, especially jazz, though my lessons included tap and ballet. My musical side was encouraged by piano lessons, musical performances, and singing. As a very young child, I would often

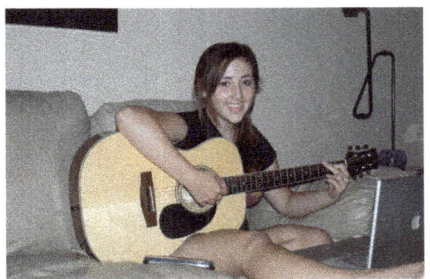

hop up on the marble coffee table and sing, "I Won't Grow Up" from the musical, Peter Pan. In those days, I dreamt of being a famous singer.

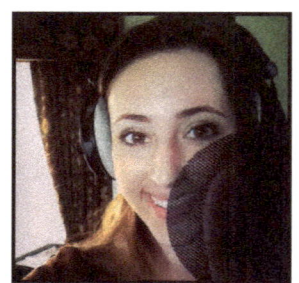

But that wasn't to be my fate—by the age of four, I was diagnosed with parvovirus B19, otherwise known as Fifth's Disease. A rather severe rash developed in my mouth, the palms of my hands, and on my feet. The pediatrician suspected coxsackievirus or Hand-Foot-and-Mouth disease, which initially angered my mother who did not realize that was a real disease and not a fabricated illness.

Somewhere along my childhood list of rash-causing illnesses, I must have contracted Roseolovirus—another perpetrator of high fevers, rashes, and eventual encephalitis. This additional viral infection wasn't recognized until later on when I tested positive for the antibodies.

With so many illnesses and so many reactions to their treatments, it is difficult to pinpoint exactly when I contracted

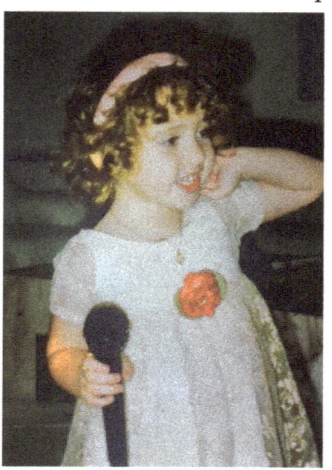

Lyme disease. Some people within the Lyme disease community that believe other vectors (such as mosquitoes or spiders) carry Lyme disease. In truth, I had been bitten by a spider at the age of three, so perhaps (though much less likely), the disease may have been transferred to my body by an arachnid, but not probable. Of course the bite was excruciating, got infected, and I was put on a new round of antibiotics.

Research is pending whether the assumption of other vectors, as ascribed by the Lyme community, is true. Much needs to be done to understand exactly how Lyme disease is transferred and by what vector.

The Center for Disease Control (CDC) describes various rashes in children. In particular, human parvovirus B19 or "Fifth Disease" is mentioned thus:

> The clinical presentation most often associated with parvovirus B19 infection is a red rash on the face, also called a "slapped cheek" rash. This is also known as Fifth Disease (or Erythema Infectiosum). This rash typically appears a few days after the fever or cold-like symptoms. It is more common in children than adults (CDC, 2024).

The symptoms sound general in nature and apparently resolve on their own. For those with weakened immunity, the CDC states there may be the long-term complications of leukemia, cancers, and other blood disorders (2024).

Obviously, the risk for additional complications to a child who has contracted any of the above is concerning. The fact that I contracted them all is overwhelming, and my history proved the CDC's suppositions correct on many levels. Interestingly, the medical experts and the CDC state that transmission of the human parvovirus B19 occurs only "through respiratory secretions and blood products [believed to] only infect humans" (Macri et al, 2023). This supposition would assume that person-to-person contact is the only means to contract human parvovirus B19. Again, medical experts have identified human parvovirus B19 as transmitted via respiratory secretions, so the probability is that I contracted that disease from a sneeze or a

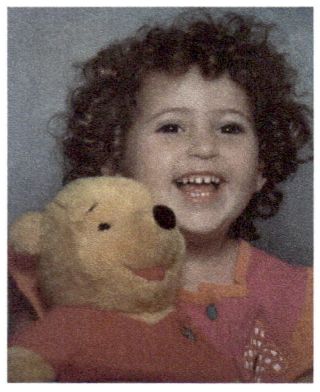

cough from an unknown carrier is legitimate.

But under atypical contexts, and given that anything is possible, including medical findings that have not yet been discovered in the transmission of disease, there is a possibility that I may be an example of such a rare circumstance, especially with the known diagnosis of human parvovirus B19 at such a young age. Currently, I test positive for existing infections of all viruses that I acquired during childhood. My body is not able to shake them. This could be from a genetic immunodeficiency or (my doctor believes) because my body is so focused fighting the Lyme disease and keeping it at bay, that it cannot cure anything else like a normal immune system does.

When evaluating the course of childhood illnesses human parvovirus B19 must be included. The result is typically a facial rash, also known as a viral exanthem that is specifically recognizable as erythema infectiosum or "Fifth Disease." The virus tends to affect children between the ages of five and fifteen, especially during warmer months (Kostolansky et al (2023). Continuing, these authors bring up the highly contagious state of an individual infected with erythema infectiosum, even after symptoms abate. Identifying the symptoms, many of which mimic flu-like illnesses, is tricky, especially for someone living with immunocompromised health.

3: Incessantly Infected

If an immunocompetent host becomes infected, there can be a range of symptoms. This can range from no symptoms to non-specific flu-like symptoms to the classic symptoms of facial rash and arthralgias (Kostolansky et al (2023).

Astute medical professionals will recognize the progression of the illness, as it advances through its various stages. These symptoms are included in the above author's findings:

Beginning symptoms of infection include:

- Fever
- Malaise
- Myalgias
- Diarrhea
- Vomiting
- Headache

After initial viremia:

- Classic erythematous malar rash involving the cheeks ("slapped-cheek rash") lasting 4-5 days.
- Surrounding oral pallor
- Joint pain
- Maculopapular rash usually on the trunk and limbs (nonpruritic or not itchy) lasting about 1 week.

While testing to identify erythema infectiosum or "Fifth Disease" is possible, the treatment is supportive care for symptoms, at this point. Possibly, management of this illness may be forthcoming in the future. One can only hope.

4:
The Physical Insult Continues

Ceclor (cefaclor) is a cephalosporin-type antibiotic commonly prescribed for broad varieties of bacterial infections, specifically those found in the ear, skin, urine, and respiratory tract. My sinus infections were not resolving, and I wasn't "growing out of it," so cefaclor was selected as the next best thing to try to combat the incessant infections that plagued my sinuses.

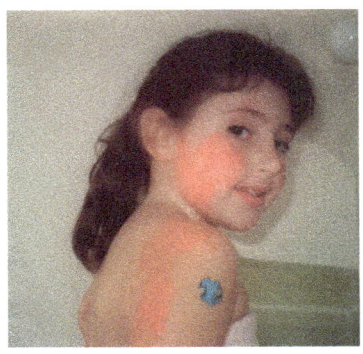 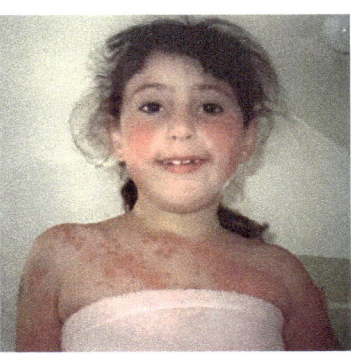

Dr. John P. Cunha (Ceclor, n.d.) consults on a lengthy list of possible side effects with this drug in RxList, an online pharmaceutical reference site. Included in this list is renal impairment, GI issues, varied and multiple types of rashes, and others. My secondary side effect was another rash, a result of developing serum sickness from a single round of the antibiotic. I looked as if I had been boiled. Apparently, I could have died from this complication—something I didn't know until recently. I was told I was lucky.

According to the CDC, a tick needs to be attached for more than 24 hours to begin filling with blood. This is the process it uses to transmit Lyme. People in the Lyme community debate about whether this is true or not. Most believe it can be transmitted more quickly than this. Because no one in my family thought the tick had attached, I did not see a doctor, keep the tick for identification, nor did I receive antibiotics (doxycycline is the preferred drug for this infection). Of course, had I received antibiotic treatment, I would have been blessed with another rash. My body could not handle any more drugs pumped into it, even those considered lifesaving antibiotics for infectious disease.

It is simply easier for physicians to dismiss the difficult diagnosis and go for one that is more familiar and treatable. Sadly, the patient suffers and lives with side effects from the trials and errors that medicine provides. Looking back now, I can see how the pieces fit. My current state of late-stage neurological Lyme disease was prepped by the diffuse and diverse use of antibiotic therapy that the medical field continued to lob at me. Nothing stuck, and I continued to suffer with a disease not yet identified.

It's important to understand Lyme disease and how that affects humans. Lyme disease (Lyme borreliosis) is a tick-borne, zoonotic disease of adults and children caused by the genospecies of the *Borrelia burgdorferi* (Radolf et al, 2021). This nasty little "bug," first associated with a black leg (deer) tick, can transfer bacterium that leads to a disease we know as Lyme disease or Lyme borreliosis. The symptoms typically associated with Lyme disease are noted as an acute illness that is responsive to treatment and manifests a systemic inflammatory response that includes a rash.

Tissue damage and symptomatology (i.e., clinical manifestations) result from the inflammatory response elicited by the bacterium and its constituents. The deposition of spirochetes into human dermal tissue generates a local inflammatory response that manifests as erythema migrans (EM), the hallmark skin lesion. If treated appropriately and early, the prognosis is excellent. However, in untreated patients, the disease may present a wide range of clinical manifestations, most commonly involving the central nervous system, joints, or heart. A small percentage (~20% to 30%) of patients may go on to develop a poorly defined fibromyalgia-like illness, post-treatment Lyme disease (PTLD) unresponsive to prolonged antimicrobial therapy (Radolf et al, 2021).

While not everyone who contracts Lyme disease is symptomatic, those who do can be overwhelmed by the symptomatology. For the few who remain unresponsive to prolonged therapy, life is altered, and their prognosis is devastating.

My experience with this nasty little bug occurred as a child while amid antibiotic therapy for various infections. I was young and still had a weakened immunity from all the antibiotics I'd been taking or perhaps the problem lies in genetic immunodeficiency. Either way, I became a perfect host for a tick.

Unfortunately, I was one of 20-30% who never fully recovered.

ACTIONS and REACTIONS

"I don't need easy… I just need possible."

~ Bethany Hamilton

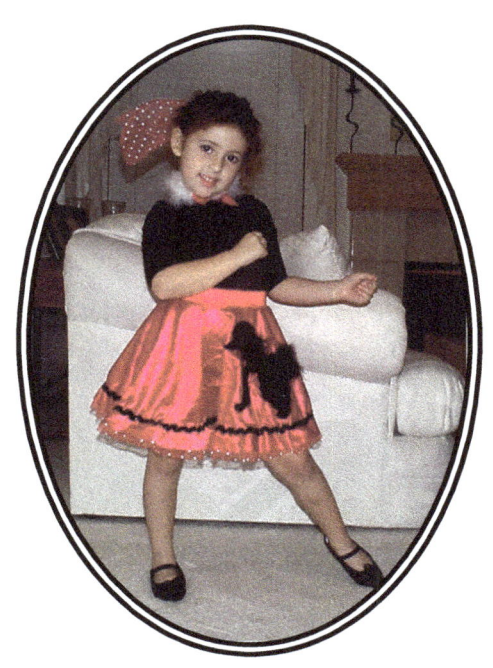

5:
Possibilities

My parents wanted me in the gifted student's program in elementary school. I cried. The long, drawn-out exams given for that program, and that I needed to pass, were daunting—especially the math exam. I had trouble focusing for extended periods of time and the thought it made me feel was dread. Believe it or not, I was somewhat quiet and very shy in school, but I had a group of good friends. I participated in Girl Scouts for a few years during this time in an effort to stay social.

Summertime was one of the best seasons in my young life. Swimming was the catalyst, which I would seek out as often as possible, testing my abilities and feeling the freedom of floating above and dipping below the surface of water that kept me buoyant. One summer day, I dove into the pool and dislocated my

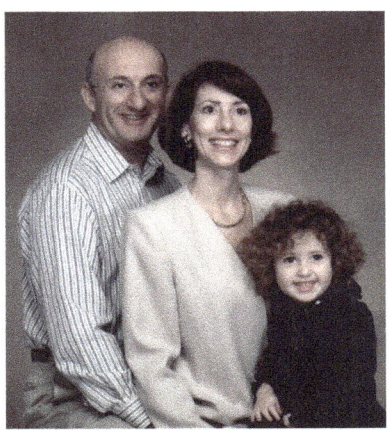

wrist, hitting my wrist on the bottom of the shallow pool. I also hit my head and jarred my neck; a detail I did not bother to tell my parents. My dad had pulled on my wrist and by the time I got to the orthopedic doctor, it had slipped back in the socket. Thankfully, I wore a waterproof cast for a month or so and still spent the summer swimming.

In third grade, I was chosen with three other students to attend a gifted student's summer camp. My teacher promised art, literature, and activities that actually sounded fun to me. As best friends, my "bestie" also attended the camp with me and thoroughly enjoyed it. This was in 2001, the year we would buy my "heart horse," *Quest Go Fancy*. A bay snowflake appendix Appaloosa Quarter horse would be my next best friend…

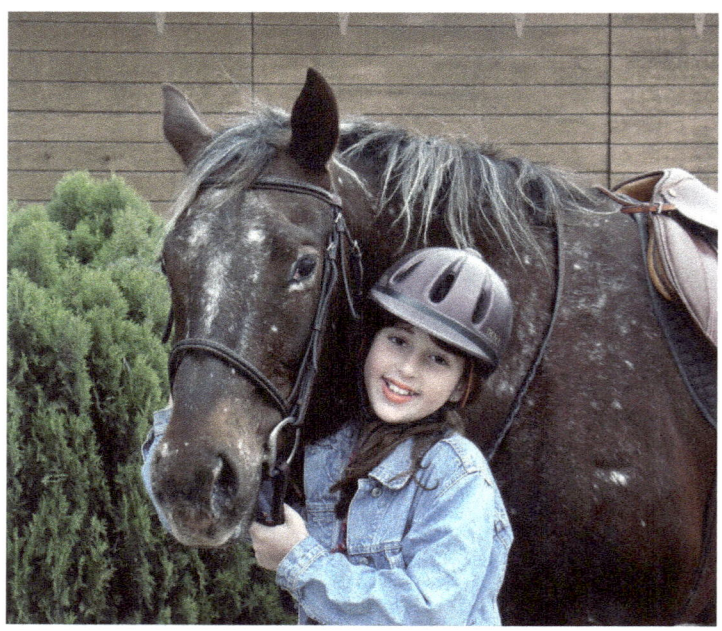

... until I lost her at the height of my illness in 2019.

5: Possibilities

In those days, the barn became my sanctuary, located on the El Toro marine base. I don't recall any ticks, but after a recent discussion with a friend, she recalls finding ticks in her horse's tail after taking him out of that barn. We also had mice in our tack shed. It is a fact that mice can carry ticks with Lyme disease. Cases have been reported, specifically on the white-footed mouse. I'm not sure if this was the type of mouse found on the marine base, something that would be of concern. Still, I don't recall ever being bitten or seeing a tick during these days, and my mom dressed me covered in long socks and riding pants most days. However, I need to be clear… it *is* possible to get Lyme disease in California.

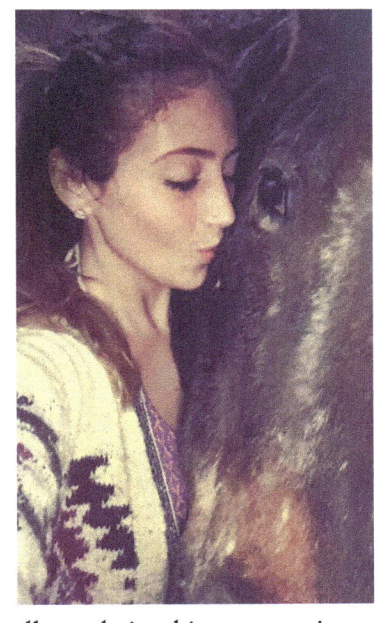

In fourth grade, I played violin. I was okay, but it wasn't something I was passionate about. Fifth grade inspired me to switch to flute, and this is where I excelled. I was chosen for honor band and played in it every year.

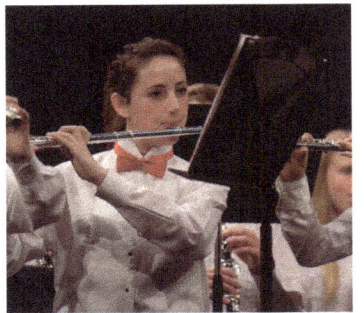

In the beginning, I loved the flute and would later advance to first chair in middle school. Band camp happened that year and I was chosen for their higher-level band with students much older than me. I took lessons with a professional. He eventually told me I played better than he did and that there was nothing left to teach me.

My spirits were high and my enthusiasm for horseback riding and music soared. The possibilities were endless. I had the world ahead of me... at least that's what I believed. My body didn't, apparently.

Controversy surrounds the diagnosis of *chronic Lyme disease* in the medical field. While some physicians support the research that demonstrates a link to the bacteria that causes Lyme disease, many medical professionals remain ambiguous as to the validity of the bacteria from a tick bite resulting in Lyme disease symptomology long-term.

Lindsay Keys (2024) provided a very interesting interview in which she discussed chronic symptoms following Lyme disease infection. In that interview, she speaks of her frustration with the CDC's lack of recognition for the disease symptoms, claiming the syndrome cannot be derived from the disease. However, bacteria are listed as a link possibly leading back to chronic symptoms. The dichotomy is maddening for those who suffer from long-term symptoms of Lyme disease. Ms. Keys continues to discuss research and scientific evidence that suggest, in some cases, Lyme disease is a persistent infection, in which short courses of antibiotics have proven not to cure humans. However, in the absence of antibiotics, the bacteria start to grow back inside the body. Ms. Keys calls this a "stop-gap measure" and brings up the need for clinical trial testing (the last clinical trial funded by the NIH was 18 years ago).

The information presented by the CDC is in direct opposition to that provided by the International Lyme and Associated Diseases Society (ILADS). For those suffering from chronic symptoms, the information offered by ILADS is invaluable and gives support to so many who suffer with chronic illness from Lyme.

The International Lyme and Associated Diseases Society (ILADS) provides its evidence-based definition of chronic Lyme disease. *Definition*: ILADS defines chronic Lyme disease (CLD) as a multisystem illness with a wide range of symptoms and/or signs that are either continuously or intermittently present for a minimum of six months. The illness is the result of an active and ongoing infection by any of several pathogenic members of the *Borrelia burgdorferi sensu lato* complex (Shor, 2019).

Certainly, physicians and other medical professionals could get on board with ILADS's efforts, continue the research into chronic symptoms' cause and effect, with the intention of identifying ways to assuage the symptoms, if not the illness.

6:
Pretty Sick Dancer

"You're too pretty to be sick."

I glanced up at my mom waiting for her response, but the doctor had more to say. His tone shifted into "adult mode" as he addressed my mother.

"Really, she's just trying to get attention."

Shocked, I waited. I knew my mother would never let this type of comment settle, and I was right.

"She's an only child. The last thing she seeks is attention," she replied.

"Well, then my recommendation is that she see a psychiatrist. At this point—"

Mom took my hand. "Let's go, sweetie." We headed for the door. "The last thing she's looking for is attention. What she needs… what we both need are answers," her last comment punctuated by the door closing to the exam room.

And so it went with several doctors, playing the same blame-game with me, suggesting my physical symptoms were in my head or that I was begging for someone to notice me. Nothing could have been further from the truth. Incessant redness and swelling to my cheeks and hands (described as a "pins-and-needles" feeling called paresthesia) spoke otherwise, but those symptoms didn't appear to be of significance to the doctors without answers.

I was only ten years old and for the next two years, my life would consist of excruciating pain, erythema and edema randomly appearing over my body, and there were no answers. The hunt for a physician who could possibly help identify what was happening to me continued… without success.

Over the course of those two years, we ruled out illness after illness. Negative tests trailed me like breadcrumbs in a fairy tale. But this was no children's story, this was a child's nightmare!

"Her results are negative for lupus," the M.D. said. We chalked that off the list.

"The tests show she doesn't have juvenile rheumatoid arthritis," another M.D. said. Check again.

Over and over again, new tests were performed along with the previous ones, according to doctors "just in case something shows up that we didn't see earlier," but everything came back negative. My reassurance: "You should be happy the tests are negative" from one of the rheumatologists. My only reaction was to cry. The tears flowed, along with my angst that this would be my life, forever. After so many years of testing and visiting specialists, we were no further than we were when the symptoms started.

We'd reached a dead-end.

All I had asked for was answers: Why am I in constant excruciating pain? Why is my immune system so bad? Why do my cheeks turn bright red and burn? Why do my hands do the same and stay mangled with pain? The only answer my young 12-year-old brain could come up with was devastating. But I had to do something… no one else could. So, I approached my mother with a solution.

"I want to quit dance."

6: Pretty Sick Dancer

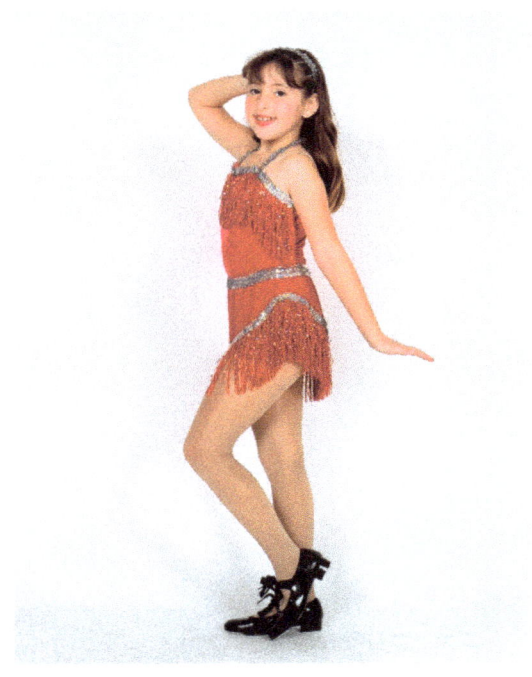

7:
Heat

"You have heat in your body," the rheumatologist said.

What does that mean exactly? I wondered, but there were no answers. "Heat" seemed to be the only response a young girl in middle-school could understand, at least that was the impression that doctor gave me. In truth, she had referred to a Chinese medicine term that meant "heat." I didn't understand it and she didn't explain it well, other than the implication that she could sense something was physically wrong.

The pain in my knee was excruciating: a 9 to 10/10 when asked for a pain scale. I'm not sure they believed me, though. Apparently, I had water on my knee—and you could see it was so, just by looking at it! My parents said this was when I first started complaining about not feeling well. It was also when the migraines hit, and my vision would disappear into a pink blob. These headaches felt as if my brain was too big for my skull. Surely something would explode. The only solution was to lie in a dark room with no light or sound for days, a cold compress over my eyes, and complete silence until the migraine passed.

I experienced so many symptoms during this time. My knees randomly gave out and I would fall, unexpectedly. I had severe exercise induce asthma—an "ice bucket" feeling in my chest is the best description I can give for how that felt. My jaw would dislocate, which meant I would miss school to spend the day with my mouth immovable, wide-open, and unable to close. The brain fog worsened, especially during tests. Floaters in my vision, dark circles under my eyes, repeated cavities (many Lyme disease patients struggle with dental issues), sensitivity to fluorescent overhead lighting in the classrooms, and more. The list goes on and on and on.

To add injury to insult, the middle school I attended was also infested with mold. I had little doubt that my Lyme symptoms flared as a result. To mitigate the mold issue, the school bought portables that were placed outdoors on campus to get the students out of the mold-infested classrooms and begin remediation. Muscle twitching, Bell's Palsy, jaw pain and stiffness, dental issues, tingling of nose, cheeks, sore throat, runny nose, blurry vision (I needed glasses but still squinted to see distances, such as the board in class), flashing lights in the corner of my eyes, plugged ears, oversensitivity to sound, ringing in both ears, sharp stomach pains (especially at sleep overs), random food aversions (stomach pain that would wax and wane with consuming pizza sauce, and chronic constipation), after-images in my visual fields, migratory pain, chemical sensitivity (such as allergies to lotions and detergents), and more.

I often cried easily over things I shouldn't have. The emotional toll was overwhelming. It's easy to see why.

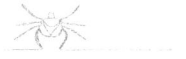

7: Heat

Symptoms of Lyme disease

Head, Face, Neck

- Unexplained hair loss (occurred with my relapse)
- **Headache, mild or severe**, seizures
- **Pressure in head**, white matter lesions in brain (MRI)
- **Twitching of facial or other muscles**
- **Facial paralysis** (**Bell's Palsy**, Horner's syndrome)
- **Tingling of nose, (tip of) tongue, cheek or facial flushing**
- **Stiff or painful neck**
- **Jaw pain or stiffness**
- **Dental problems**
- **Sore throat**, clearing throat a lot, **phlegm**, **hoarseness, runny nose**

Eyes/Vision

- Double or **blurry vision**
- **Increased floating spots**
- **Pain in eyes, or swelling around eyes**
- **Oversensitivity to light**
- **Flashing lights**, peripheral waves or phantom images in corner of eyes

Ears/Hearing

- Decreased hearing in one or both ears, **plugged ears**
- **Buzzing in ears**
- **Pain in ears, oversensitivity to sounds**
- **Ringing in one or both ears (tinnitus)**
- Digestive and Excretory Systems
- Diarrhea

- **Constipation**
- **Irritable bladder** (trouble starting, **stopping**) or interstitial cystitis
- **Upset stomach (nausea or pain)** or GERD (gastroesophageal reflux)

Musculoskeletal System

- **Bone pain, joint pain or swelling**, carpal tunnel syndrome
- **Stiffness of joints, back, neck**, tennis elbow
- **Muscle pain or cramps, (Fibromyalgia)**

Respiratory and Circulatory Systems

- **Shortness of breath, can't get full/satisfying breath, cough**
- **Chest pain or rib soreness**
- **Night sweats or unexplained chills**
- **Heart palpitations**, arrythmia or extra beats
- Endocarditis, heart blockage

Neurologic System

- **Tremors or unexplained shaking**
- **Burning or stabbing sensations in the body**
- **Fatigue, Chronic Fatigue Syndrome, weakness, peripheral neuropathy,** or **partial paralysis**
- **Pressure in the head**
- **Numbness in body, tingling, pinpricks**
- **Poor balance, dizziness, difficulty walking**
- **Increased motion sickness**
- **Light-headedness, wooziness**

7: Heat

Psychological Well-being

- **Mood swings, irritability**, bi-polar disorder (a later symptom in my case)
- **Unusual depression**
- **Disorientation (getting or feeling lost)**
- Feeling as if you are losing your mind (a later symptom in my case)
- **Over-emotional reactions, crying easily**
- **Too much sleep, or insomnia**
- **Difficulty falling or staying asleep**
- Narcolepsy, sleep apnea
- **Panic attacks, anxiety**

Mental Capability

- **Memory loss (short or long term)**
- **Confusion, difficulty thinking**
- **Difficulty with concentration or reading**
- **Going to the wrong place**
- **Speech difficulty (slurred or slow)**
- **Difficulty finding commonly used words**
- Stammering speech
- **Forgetting how to perform simple tasks**

Reproduction and Sexuality

- Loss of sex drive
- Sexual dysfunction
- **Unexplained menstrual pain, irregularity**
- **Unexplained breast pain**, discharge
- Testicular or **pelvic pain**

General Well-being

- Phantom smells
- **Unexplained weight gain** or loss
- **Extreme fatigue**
- **Swollen glands or lymph nodes**
- **Unexplained fevers** (high or **low grade**)
- **Continual infections** (**sinus**, kidney (later on), eye, etc.)
- **Symptoms seem to change, come and go**
- **Pain migrates (moves) to different body parts**
- Early on, experienced a "flu-like" illness, after which you have not since felt well (maybe? Don't remember)
- **Low body temperature**
- **Allergies or chemical sensitivities**
- Increased effect from alcohol and possible worse hangover symptoms (later on, in college)

*Physical symptoms I experienced personally are listed in bold

During this time, my teachers would allow me use of my lunchtime to finish tests, which gave me additional time to finish. At this time, I begged to be home-schooled because I felt so horrible. There were days I would feel so awful at school, I would go to the nurse and ask to go home. My pediatrician told my mom that I "was faking it." Sadly, she didn't know what to believe (I don't blame her). Finally, the school set up a meeting with my middle school counselor and my mother. My mom voiced her distress at having been told to "keep her in school" and expressed her confusion about what to believe. Luckily, the school counselor admonished my mom to listen to me, stating, "If Kaitlyn says she doesn't feel well, believe her"

This was the turning point for my parents who quickly got on board. How thankful I am for this school counselor!

7: Heat

I wasn't home-schooled, but after this "ah-ha" experience, my mom allowed me to stay home on my "flared" days. To support my family and my success in my education, my teachers made packets that allowed me to complete my work at home until I was well enough to return. This permitted me to stay in regular school.

Unfortunately, this was not the way for a teenager to spend her days.

Someone suggested acupuncture, at that point. I was desperate for any help I could get, so we began acupuncture. It helped a little bit with the pain and even the fatigue. But the suffering was not over… I guess that was because there was "heat" in my body. I also frequently visited the chiropractor for my extremely stiff and painful neck. He also adjusted my hips, which felt like they would go out of place and cause me to limp. The chiropractor would often suggest that my atlas (a bone in my neck) was out of place, which would trigger migraines.

"Dad! Mom!" I could barely contain my 12-year-old excitement. "You gotta see this. It's on TV right now. They're talking about a girl who has my same problems!"

I wasn't sure they'd heard me, so I hollered again, not moving my eye from the TV screen for fear I'd miss something important! "DAD!"

That time, they'd heard me and came running. I'm sure mom thought I had broken a bone or something serious. "What in the world?"

"Watch! Watch this! That's Jaqueline. She has the same thing I have. Look! She's just like me. I'm not the only one."

The "ah-ha" moment came while watching *Mystery Diagnosis* on TV. The episode was called "The Stabbing Sensation" and featured the story of Jaqueline Spar. I was only 12 but the truth that I was finally *seen* hit me like a brick. It was a revelation for me and my parents. Through the Spar family's advocacy, I learned I was not the only youth suffering from unexplained, debilitating symptoms such as those. That single TV show changed my life and my parents' perspective. Finally, there was hope and I was not alone.

Unexplained symptoms, such as shooting leg pain, headaches, upper respiratory, rashes, and inflammation are all indicative of Lyme disease. One mother described her daughter's symptoms (that included many of those mentioned above) as debilitating, stating, "…her hands became gnarled and she could no longer walk" (Griffin, 2011). Like my experience, Jacqueline Spar suffered from undiagnosed Lyme disease and sought answers. Her mother, Stephanie, describes her daughter's experience as, "Her life basically stopped. At the worst, she wasn't walking or talking and was mentally incoherent" (Griffin 2011)—almost an exact duplication of my symptoms.

The CDC lists the following symptoms that include those experienced by Jacqueline Spar and me. Those symptoms are listed below and can be found on the CDC's website: (https://www.cdc.gov/lyme/signs-symptoms/index.html):

- "Bull's-eye" rash
- **Fever**
- **Facial paralysis**
- Irregular heartbeat

- Arthritis

Later symptoms also included on the same CDC website include:

- **Severe headaches** and **neck stiffness**
- **Additional rashes**
- **Facial palsy**
- **Severe joint pain and swelling**, **particularly in the knees** and other **large joints**
- **Intermittent pain in tendons, muscles, joints, bones**
- **Palpitations** or irregular heartbeat (attributed to Lyme carditis)
- **Dizziness and shortness of breath**
- Spinal cord inflammation
- **Inflammation of the brain**
- **Nerve pain**
- **Numbness/tingling of the hands or feet**

*Physical symptoms I experienced personally are listed in bold

The list is impressive and is one that needs to be taken seriously. Had the physicians done so, my outcome (and likely Jacqueline's) may have been different. Unfortunately, the process of identifying Lyme disease is often a result of ruling out other illnesses. This takes time and astute observation of victims, their families, and the medical professionals who assume care of Lyme disease patients. Not knowing the underlying causes of these types of symptoms proves difficult at best, and time is not on the side of the victim. Identification of the disease in its early stages is often the key to a successful outcome. Unfortunately, that is not always possible for most.

Most recently, the CDC has expanded its search to identify and treat Lyme disease. However, the burden often falls to the victim and family members. Per the CDC website (see above):

Seek medical attention if you observe any of these symptoms and have recently had a tick bite, live in an area known for Lyme disease, or have recently traveled to an area where Lyme disease occurs.

The goal of this book is to support those who find themselves in similar situations as myself (and others) by providing my story and the subsequent information gathered as a result of my suffering in hopes that others can avoid the same aftermath.

8:
"Butterfly" Symptoms

The pain I experienced throughout my body spread, increasing in intensity until I, like Jacqueline Spar, was unable to move on occasion (see YouTube Mystery Diagnosis Lyme disease, first broadcast in 2008, now available via Clairizio, G. 2016). My days were spent seeking opinions from dozens of specialists, none of whom could provide answers.

Around this time, a butterfly rash spread across the bridge of my nose and cheeks, a classic symptom (malar rash) of autoimmune diseases and bacterial infections from Lyme disease. Still, no one recognized this as resulting from a tick bite.

So, at age twelve, I took matters in my own hands. Seeking answers the only way I knew how, I went to the internet and began a long search for symptoms of Lyme disease. Fortunately for me, a Canadian site (CanLyme—the Canadian Lyme Disease Foundation) provided a list that I printed off and handed to my parents, along with tests and instructions on *how to convince your doctor to test you.* This was significant because I counted 46 to 48 out of 52 symptoms from the checklist that I had experienced at that time. I was convinced that this was the illness I had been suffering from. All of this information was placed in a teal-colored folder and taken to my primary care physician.

"Please run the tests," I begged. "You can see for yourself that I have almost every single symptom listed here." I pointed to the Canadian list of indicators.

He agreed and ran the standard Western Blot test.

"The results are indeterminate," he replied later.

"What does that mean? What does it mean!" I began to panic a little.

My mother stepped into the conversation. "What can you do for her then, with an indeterminate finding?"

The doctor glanced at the results in his hands and paused. "Well," he finally spoke, "I feel comfortable enough to try antibiotics with this result. I think a course of Doxycycline won't hurt."

A month went by, and my symptoms had improved, enough that I was able to go on our annual family trip to Missouri. The pain had dissipated enough that I hardly noticed it at all, and the nausea that accompanied the antibiotic seemed minimal compared to the relief I experienced. After that month and the course of Doxycycline was completed, the pain returned. Discouragement returned as well. Mom called the doctor explaining that my symptoms recurred as soon as I stopped taking the antibiotics.

"Let's give it another go," he said, and prescribed another month's worth of Doxy for me. Again, no pain. No other symptoms, as well. I was certain that this second month of antibiotic treatment had done the trick, and this time would be the end of my Lyme journey.

Unfortunately, it was only the beginning.

8: "Butterfly" Symptoms

Little is said about chronic Lyme disease, and its link back to the initial illness. In fact, the Center for Disease Control (CDC) does not recognize chronic Lyme disease. They maintain that chronic symptoms from Lyme disease are actually a syndrome that cannot be derived from the disease. The bacterium is listed on the CDC website (2024) as linked to *possibly leading to* chronic symptoms. Fortunately, the CDC does not entirely dismiss the concept of a syndrome development, termed posttreatment Lyme disease symptoms or syndrome or PTLDS. From the same site (2024):

Although PTLDS is generally more common in women and in persons who have a difficult early disease course, the underlying causes are not well understood, and biomarkers to identify patients at risk for such outcomes are lacking. Thus, treatment strategies are symptom-based and often ineffective, leaving patients and physicians in a quandary about how to restore health.

Perhaps this view of a *possible syndrome* led to the reluctance of physicians in identifying and treating anything other than symptoms, even with testing that suggested positive results in patients with tick bite history.

9:
Gym Time

"Let's get you signed up for a gym."

My parents were adamant that increased exercise would help with the sudden weight gain. I felt pretty good, not great, but better by the time 8th grade started, so I was hopeful that maybe one more attempt at getting healthier would help. Maybe a gym membership would do the trick.

"Ten pounds is a lot to lose. You'll really have to make an effort."

I agreed with my parents' reasoning, mainly because I had been so embarrassed at school when the students were asked to step on the scales in P.E. Not expecting the results, everyone discovered I weighed at least ten pounds more than the other girls. It was humiliating and working out at a gym was my parents' best solution.

My 13th year was tough, not only because of "teenage issues" that accompanied Jr. High aged kids, but also because of the weight that felt more like exaggerated embarrassment, and my health. Like most young girls that age, I decided I wanted to be a cheerleader and began taking tumbling and cheering lessons. This was problematic on my still very painful joints. I worked just as hard as the other girls, but it

Kaitlyn Oleinik

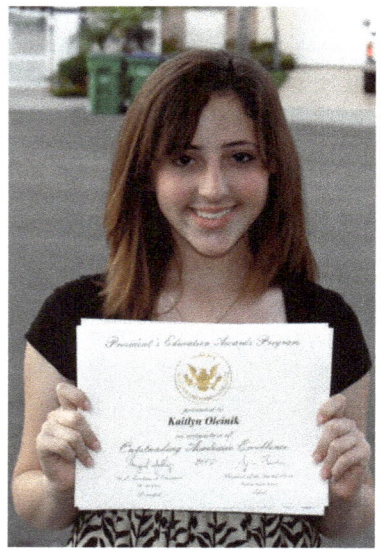

would take a longer time to be able to learn the tricks—mostly because of the pain (and lack of synchronization with my brain). Unfortunately, my joints would dislocate during tricks like a back handspring. The entire process and effort involved made little sense, especially the pain I suffered in doing so, but I was determined.

Soon, it became a reality that cheer team wasn't in my future for that first year. Mostly, the fear of a back handspring on their thin, hard mats prevented me from going all-out. I was certain it wouldn't end well. Playing it safe left me without much injury, except for a broken heart at the realization I wouldn't make the team. I graduated middle school earning the President's Education award for "Outstanding Academic Excellence."

As the year progressed, so did my weight gain. High school began with few friends—some of the old ones remained loyal but I had trouble making new friends. This proved difficult, and my ability to adjust to high school life as a teenager was affected.

Adding to the problems at school, I continued to compare my eating habits with my peers. No matter what I ate, I continued to gain weight (at one point reaching 177 pounds). Joining a weight loss program seemed to be the next option and so I became a dedicated member of one of the programs. The weight finally came off but the consequences followed.

Eating disorders are a common problem for those suffering with Lyme disease. This was true for me, as I began to binge and purge, developing bulimia.

My newest fear: gaining weight

Dr. Daniel Kinderlehrer, MD speaks of the critical nature of eating disorders associated with Lyme disease. In his blog entitled, *Introducing Lyme and Eating Disorders* (2024), Dr. Kinderlehrer acknowledges the numerous reviews found in medical literature that document neuropsychiatric conditions associated with Lyme disease, stating "most of them include the general category of 'eating disorders'." He continues, "Anorexia nervosa is increasingly common and it is serious—it has the highest mortality of any "psychiatric" disorder" (Kinderlehrer, 2024).

The struggle that follows the symptomatology of Lyme disease is real. Victims manifest differently, but the patterns are similar—one of which is eating disorders.

I was no exception.

At that time, I knew nothing about bands for Lyme disease, and I didn't ask to physically see the results when they were available a few years earlier. I wish more than anything I had a copy of that test. My best educated guess is that the results came back for me as multiple positive bands, but not enough to be considered "CDC qualified positive," meaning five or more bands per test. By all accounts, my test likely showed that I had been exposed to Lyme bacteria.

Had I known this, the outcome may have been different.

10:
Brain Fog

Speak!

The teacher had written this on my grade sheets again. It wasn't my fault, really. I just didn't fit in, and that affected my ability to socialize, to respond, and to "speak up" during class in high school.

Growing up in Southern California, it was cool to be 115 pounds with beach-blonde hair and cool clothes to match. I had the clothes, but I did not look like the typical California girl. As a result, (in combination with crippling social anxiety) I had trouble making new friends.

Part of the problem was my brain fog (from Lyme disease) during this time. Social stress and what felt like increased inflammation in my head would shut me down, and I could not think of anything to say—at all. The result led to a situation in which I would almost go mute. Mostly, this happened in social and academic settings such as the seminars we had to do for AP English classes.

Rarely, if ever, would I talk about my problem, and I definitely didn't confide in any of my high school teachers about the issues I was having with health and social interaction. In retrospect, I probably should have.

Absenteeism was a pattern that followed me throughout high school, as I continued to miss long stretches of school, getting sick for one to two months at a time. My self-esteem took another turn for the worse, and I began to feel very self-conscious and shy. Still, I was able to keep up my grades and came home with mostly A's and B's.

When I entered accelerated math, I had trouble concentrating and noticed a shift in my performance, compared to my other grades.

"She's not doing well," my teacher reported to my mother over the phone.

"Well, what's going on?" mom replied.

There was a slight pause. "I'm not sure. But she isn't retaining anything and her grades are beginning to suffer because of it. I'm not sure she is comprehending what's being taught… or maybe she just isn't listening."

My mom took me to a psychiatrist in hopes of finding an answer. That came after extensive testing with a diagnosis of Attention Deficit Disorder (ADD).

"We can handle this with medication for treatment," the psychiatrist suggested.

Immediately, I was prescribed Adderall. At the ripe old age of

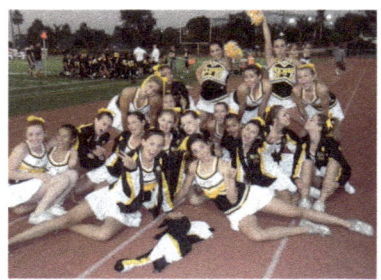
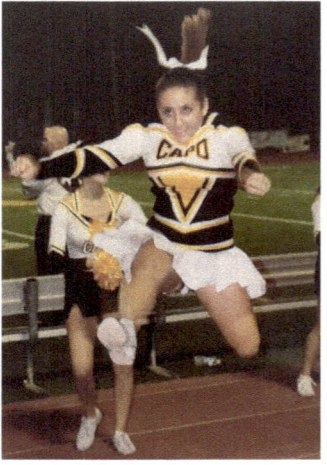

High school cheer team

10: Brain Fog

fifteen, the effects were significant. I felt different and would lose track of time. Suddenly, I would hyper-focus on one activity for hours at a time. My anxiety increased. This was not the way a young teenage girl should feel—numbed out and fearful. So, I elected not to take it every day.

Cheer came around again about that time.

"I'm going to give it another go," I told my parents. They supported me and this time, I made the cheer team. Life was manageable for a while.

My period stopped for a month, accompanied by a sharp pain in my pelvis, driving me to fall to the floor. Therein followed another visit to the emergency department. While there, the ER doctor asked if I had been making myself throw up (an interesting but astute observation). But they found a small amount of fluid in my pelvic area and believed an ovarian cyst might have ruptured, causing the excruciating pain. I realized the detriment my eating disorder had on my body and stopped the bulimic behavior after this—something my therapist and treatment centers had said is very rare to do (to stop on one's own, but the ER visit scared me straight).

I graduated with a 3.5 GPA and qualified for an honors tassel. Due to my many absences, it wasn't ordered in time. Because it took longer to get my work submitted (to get the GPA and to qualify) they had already ordered the tassel, which was the wrong color combination. Mine was black and yellow (it wasn't supposed to have any black in it at all and I considered cutting all of the black strings out—I probably should have, thinking about it now). When I asked for a yellow tassel, the school said it was too late to order one and pointed out that if I had missed only seven additional days of school, I wouldn't have been able to graduate. "So, you should just be happy you're graduating at all!"

Kaitlyn Oleinik

Even though I would graduate with honors, they hassled me for absences that that could not be controlled due to illness.

Often, mom wrote notes excusing me for lunch to allow me to spend that time with my horse, instead of attempting to make new friends at the school lunch break. In truth, my horse was my therapy during this time.

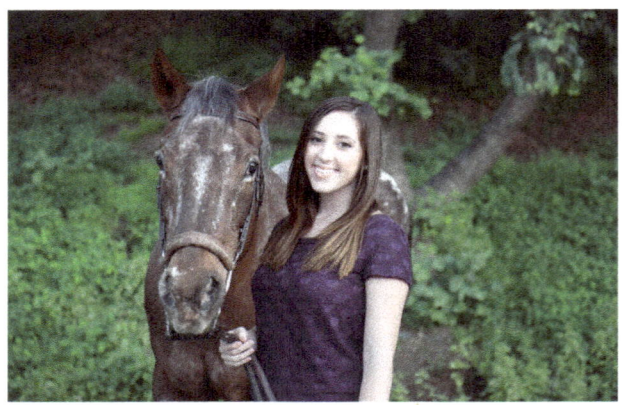

More Than Just an Education

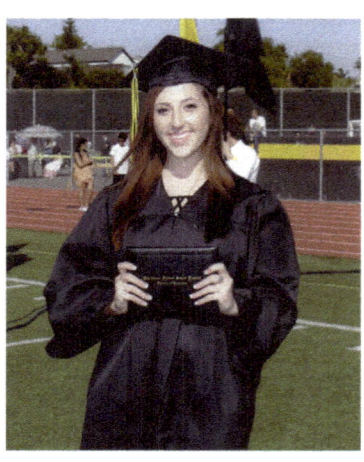

11:
Back to School

Then came college.

"I would recommend only four classes to begin with."

I looked at the counselor who returned my gaze over the glasses perched on her nose. She knit her fingers together and forced a smile meant to intimidate me into agreeing with her.

"But aren't full-time studies classified as five classes, not four?" I asked.

The counselor nodded and shuffled some papers on her desk. "Yes, that's correct. You will still be able to graduate on time. I recommend all students start slowly." Apparently, this was her recommendation for all students, provided they could still graduate on time. I never opened up about any of my issues to my teachers or counselors.

So, I took the recommended four classes and made the best of it.

Part of that "best" was finding a best friend and meeting my would-be boyfriend, both before school started. Finally, I had a group of friends. By now, I had become reliant on Adderall, particularly in dealing with fatigue and getting homework done. Focusing was difficult, and writing papers on a timeline was nearly impossible.

It felt as if there were less hours in the day, for me more than for anyone else. How my peers would get all of their homework done, have time to socialize, and then party three to four nights a week was unexplainable. My energy level wouldn't allow it and I considered myself lucky with only one night out per week.

I remember one night lying in bed at 9:00 pm, exhausted, ready to end the day. A conversation was happening in the next room between my roommate and her friend. Most of their conversation was garbled, except one comment that sounded rather clear despite their low voices.

"In bed at nine p.m.? What's wrong with her?"

That one comment stayed with me.

Often, a friend would come over to watch movies on the television with me, and I would fall asleep. It wasn't much of an interaction, but it was something. At this point, I was grateful for anything, and friends who stayed loyal to me during my college days were important.

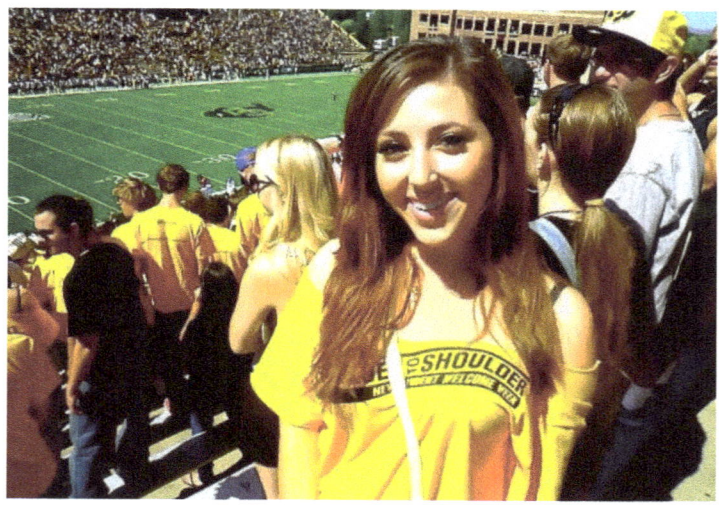

In college, my weight stabilized. I dropped from 150 pounds to 135 pounds and felt happy with it. For the first time in a long time, I was content with my body. I got sick a couple times during that year, strep throat being one of the illnesses that plagued me, but I did not miss the month-long stretch of school that had occurred while living at home.

While at Boulder, my writing and class work were praised, and I quickly noticed that the professors took more of an interest in my success than did the teachers in high school or middle school. Even though the snow made my joints ache, and I had trouble maneuvering in the snow from one side of the campus to the other within the allocated 10 to 15 minutes between classes, college became a bitter-sweet time for me.

Often, I would find myself in tears. Sadness seemed to follow me around the campus, and my best friend could do little to help—she had her own personal trauma and dealt with depression.

"Turn it up," I told her one day.

"Done!" she replied as she cranked the radio on her dashboard. The mountains seemed to lift our spirits as we climbed higher in the peaks. Never mind the twisting roads, we needed the fresh mountain air and a breather from school. I glanced at my best friend and realized that this was the first time I felt like I had someone who fully understood me. She was a sister from different parents and I loved her like family.

That same day, we had climbed about as high as we could on our drive and decided to stop, take in the views, and just enjoy the moment. I figured this was the best time to tell her.

"I think he's the one."

She glanced at me and a slow grin spread across her face. "*The* one?"

I nodded. "I'm falling in love with him… I know it. He's from a good family with good values."

"My kind of guy," she replied, wistfully.
"Mine too."

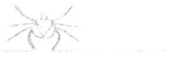

Trauma materializes in many different forms, and its victims wear just as many disguises to cover it up. Unfortunately, for many, the mask that is mental health hides the face that is a tick-borne illness. Medical professionals typically see the issue as the symptom—mental illness while the cause is often ignored. While mental illness is truly a devastating disease, there exist causes that lie deeper than the mental illness itself. Lyme disease is one of those causes of mental illness.

Research conducted at the Columbia University Irving Medical Center and the Copenhagen Research Centre for Mental Health identified the correlation between Lyme disease and mental illness.

For patients, these ongoing and sometimes debilitating symptoms can erode their quality of life, potentially leading to depression, anxiety, and other mental health issues. But over the past few decades, researchers have also determined that the tick-borne infection itself, along with related inflammatory and other physiological effects, may directly cause mental health disorders. One recent study found that patients who received a hospital diagnosis of Lyme disease had a 28% higher rate of mental disorders and were twice as likely to have attempted suicide postinfection than individuals without a Lyme diagnosis (American Psychological Association, 2022).

It is high time the medical profession looks beyond symptoms, such as mental illness, to determine the *cause* of the disease that manifests as symptoms.

11: Back to School

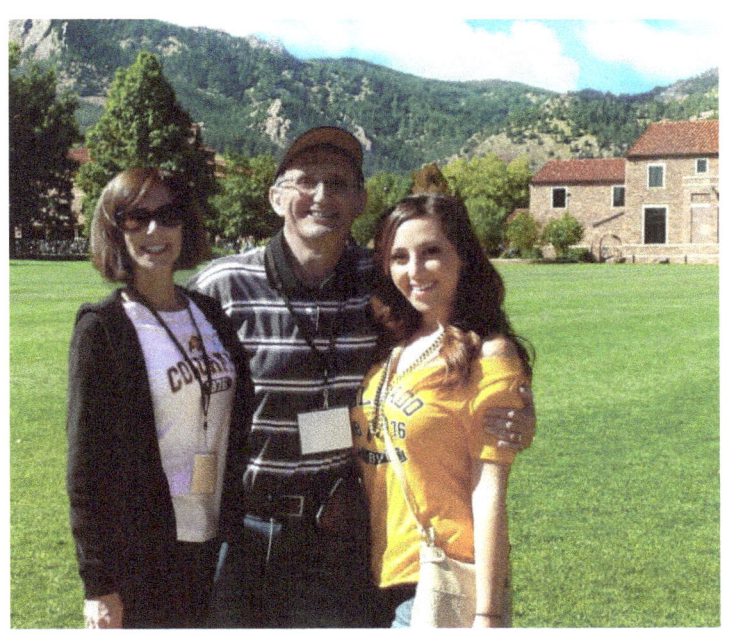

12:
Relationships

"I'm just not ready to be in this deep." He couldn't look me in the eyes, which was probably a good thing because mine were filled with tears.

"I get it," I said.

"No really, it isn't you. I'm just messed up. I'm just not ready for another relationship after my last one. It was bad, Kaitlyn."

"I really get it."

He paused. "You're amazing. And I'm probably making the next biggest mistake of my life by walking away from you. But I'm just not... you know."

I couldn't say anything more.

I should've listened. It would've saved me a lot of heart ache. But I was determined to show him he could trust me. Still, he decided the best thing was to break up that summer. I'm certain it's because he didn't trust me (or anyone else) to do a long distance relationship.

I cried every day that summer. Every. Single. Day.

My self-worth was as low as it had ever been. Even though I kept telling myself *you deserve someone who picks you every day*, the heartache continued. It would take a while for me to understand what that meant exactly.

His friends were hyper-focused on partying, drinking, and even using drugs. That was not my gig. So, I stayed quiet and tried to remain invisible around his friends. Regardless, I found it hard to relate to them. Eventually, this had become a source of tension in our relationship, driving a deeper wedge between us.

My sophomore year was supposed to be the year I lived on campus with a friend. Of course, she bailed on me at the last second and took a spot that had opened up in a house with our mutual friends. So, I lived on campus alone. Sadly, my best friend didn't do well at Boulder and had to move back home to attend a community college. I was gutted. In the meantime, another close friend, someone I trusted, decided to leave campus, as well, to attend an entirely different school.

That year started with no friends, living alone, and managing a severe bladder infection. Initially, it was believed the symptoms were due to food poisoning. I would vomit in between classes and sometimes enroute to class. It took a while to figure out what was wrong.

Drama commenced that year, as if the first few weeks weren't enough. The phone call came unexpectedly.

"Hey… um… I want another chance to work things out between us."

I didn't know how to respond. "You want what?"

"Look, I made a mistake. We were good together and I just didn't get it. I want to try again." His voice sounded shaky at first but the tenderness I heard got to me.

"Why? What about the long-distance relationship thing? It's still there and still a problem, isn't it?" I asked, feeling hopeful.

"Not a problem anymore. At least, I don't think it will be. Please, Kaitlyn. Give me another chance."

I agreed. After all, I loved him… and he was *the one*.

12: Relationships

Hope is a powerful force that can drive people to make wise… and not so wise decisions. Those who suffer from the ravages of Lyme disease understand how fragile but commanding hope can be. We live with the delicate balance between the hope for heath and finding that hope dashed as another symptom raises its ugly head to make us ill.

Included in wellness and effective healing is empowerment of the affected individual and hopefulness. The mental health that surrounds a state of being self-empowered, involved in planning, respected in opinion and thought, and viewed as a valued member of the collaborative team brings a positive experience to the patient and fosters the healing sentiment of hope. This encourages a forward-thinking state and is considered a therapeutic dynamic that aids in a positive recovery process (Melville, 2025). Research supports Melville's theory:

Hope has been considered to be a positive attribute for achieving a better quality of life, especially in patients with chronic disease. Previous research has reported that hope was associated with health indicators, such as coping, self-esteem, and quality of life (Mardhiyah et al, 2020).

The direct and indirect influence of hope on an individual's life (particularly the youth) leads to a positive quality of life.

13:
Gaslighting

I couldn't trust him—in my gut, I knew it.

He would lie to me, small lies that I would catch, and it was just enough to open my eyes and pique that pit in my stomach, warning me that something was off. Sadly, the whole thing brought about panic attacks and days when I couldn't stop crying, especially when he would go out alone with his friends.

"I just want to go with you." My request was met with his brow furrowed and his eyes narrowed to slits.

"I told you. This isn't something that dates go to. Just me and my posse," he quipped, but there was anger hidden in his voice.

"But…"

"No! I said, NO!"

His temper flared quickly and our conversation escalated into a fight too quickly. He was hiding something, I knew it. Behind my gut warning me of his covert behavior, I still feared he would break up with me and that felt worse than being lied to. It was obvious that I had nothing to compare a bad relationship to—I'd never experienced a healthy one—so fear felt normal.

Friendships with others during this time took a backseat to everything and I didn't make friends with any of the girls in my dorm as a result. They were all freshman and the effort was too great, so I let that part of my life go. Most days, I ate breakfast alone. It left me very isolated and feeling abandoned. In an effort to associate with my boyfriend's buddies, I wasted my time. Statistics was on my class roster and, as it turned out, I had a wonderful tutor that got me through the course. That was a positive!

My junior year arrived and I continued to lose friends who would decide that CU Boulder wasn't for them. Most roommates commented that I was an introvert and called me "The most elusive roommate of the bunch." They were probably right, since most of my time was spent in my room resting and doing homework. It simply took more effort to keep up with school, so resting had become a necessary tool for success.

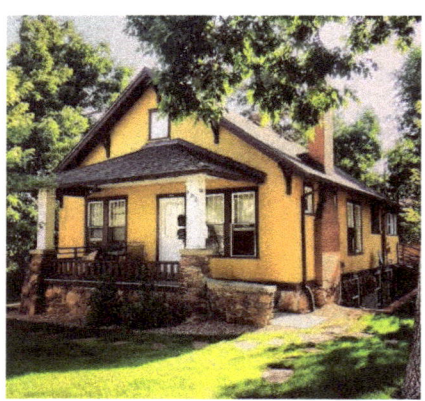

In September of 2013, Boulder flooded. We lived in the basement level of a house. My room got it the worst. Mold crept in after the water damage and my entire closet, my shoes, my clothes, everything I owned had mold on it—even the

13: Gaslighting

closet wall, which was full of water. As the paint peeled, I would push on the wall and feel water bounce, trapped between the sheetrock and the very thin layer of paint.

Soon, I developed a cough. My roommates noticed my cough.

"Girl, you are always coughing. Is the air okay for you? Maybe you should get that checked out!"

The landlord found out and questioned my health. "We're concerned about reports that you're coughing a lot. What's going on? Have you seen a doctor about that?"

"I've got Lyme disease and can't be around mold. There's mold everywhere from the flooding."

"I see. Well, I've had it tested and the mold in your apartment isn't considered the toxic kind."

I couldn't believe what I was hearing. "But my room is covered in mold and I can't be around *any* mold, of *any kind*."

The landlord looked at me and the smile dropped from her face. "I understand. But we had it tested and it's not toxic. Everyone in the neighborhood has the same problem and we need to step up as neighbors. I have to help them out first. You'll be fine."

"This is urgent. I don't think you understand how serious this is for me."

"Really, Kaitlyn. You should be thankful it's only mold. Other people in Boulder have it much worse than you do," the landlord turned on her heel and walked away. "You'll be fine."

Once again, I was not a priority. Even with the money I was paying to live in her damaged home, she couldn't be bothered to fix the mold issue. Obviously, the lady had no idea of how serious mold can be with Lyme disease. I should have listened to my gut feeling on this, as well, and moved into a hotel until the situation was handled properly. But I did not yet understand the severity of mold's effect on Lyme disease.

Unfortunately, ignorance compounded the issue as we did everything wrong to treat the mold, including spraying it with bleach. Since learning that doing so releases the spores into the air, making it difficult to breathe, bleach is no longer a go-to for dealing with mold. Even the dehumidifier failed to clear up the issues with inhaling mold and water—even with multiple daily draining.

It seems no coincidence that with the exposure to mold, my anxiety and panic attacks would spiral out of control. My boyfriend had no empathy or patience for it. The chronic anxiety just made him angry.

Symptoms included, not only the mental and emotional stress accompanying anxiety and PTSD, but also lethargy. Adderall was the physicians' go-to for treatment and I soon became so completely reliant on the drug that I was unable to do any tasks without it, especially homework.

Once, while pulling an "all-nighter" to finish an assignment, I found myself spiraling into a full-blown panic attack due to my inability to think of anything to write. My mind was completely blank. The assignment was due and the only thing I could produce was absolute panic.

"I need to go to the ER." My voice quivered as I spoke and fought back tears, waiting for my boyfriend's response.

"Why?"

"It's my heart. Something is wrong with it… I can feel it. It's not beating right."

Just then, I heard my own voice scream in my head. It was my first auditory hallucination. I don't know what triggered it but glancing at the mold still growing on my bedroom wall, seeing either that black entity or the Adderall sitting on my dresser crawled into my brain.

Had I realized what was going on, I would have recognized this as an early sign of auditory hallucinations.

13: Gaslighting

"I think I'm dying," I whispered into the phone's receiver.

"I'll be right over," he said and moments later, picked me up and drove me to the nearest emergency department.

The wait for my results was interminable! Even with the medications and IVs, the panic continued to rise. I had never had a panic attack this strong before, so I knew it was more than just my anxiety. *Something* definitely was wrong with my heart… with my body!

"The tests are negative. There's nothing wrong," he said smiling. I noticed his teeth matched the color of his lab coat and my stomach heaved. "Maybe you hyperventilated and felt like you were going to pass out from the anxiety of it all."

I could only stare at the doctor, who smiled dismissively at me. The nurse had already removed my IV and was preparing me for discharge. "I'm pretty sure that's not it. My heart…"

The doctor patted my shoulder, and I noticed his fingernails were as pristine as his smile. I sighed and he walked out of the room. *It's not a panic attack*, I thought to myself and blinked back tears as I dressed.

This was the first experience in Colorado and a quick education on dismissive doctors.

"Gaslighting" is a kitsch term that evolved from George Cukor's 1944 film *Gaslight*, starring Ingrid Bergman and Charles Boyer. The story follows the manipulation and mental abuse of a woman (Bergman) by her husband (Boyer) in an attempt to alter her perception of reality, eventually making her believe she is crazy. This scenario, while fictional in the film, unfortunately is common and occurs as a form of abuse to its victims. The damage is real and lasting, as Sweet (2019) points out.

Kaitlyn Oleinik

Gaslighting is linked to insidious patterns of control, in which women are denied mobility, access to their social networks, and institutional help. Gaslighting strategies that draw on women's institutional vulnerabilities are especially effective at keeping women isolated and entrapped: abusers manipulate women's fear of and lack of credibility in institutions to make them seem "crazy" and to control them further.

When a specific outcome is desired of another individual, nefarious gaslighting methods can be used to manipulate the targeted individual and control is obtained by the abuser. When this occurs in an institutional setting, such as was my case with the doctor, hindsight would suggest the doctor did not have answers or solutions to the problems I presented. As a result, the physician's ego was tested and the unfortunate result was to gaslight the patient (me) instead of admitting lack.

Gaslighting is common in domestic violence situations, preventing women from accessing resources… analysis shows, gaslighting can amplify the dangers already present in abused women's lives (Sweet, 2019).

It is incumbent upon medical professionals to recognize when ego gets in the way of care for their patient, especially when the patient expresses concern and the tendency is to counter with, "There's nothing wrong with you," leading to a gaslighting (abusive) response.

Post traumatic stress disorder (PTSD) can be the outcome of this type of abuse.

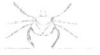

Post-traumatic stress disorder (PTSD) is comprised of three symptom clusters including (1) re-experiencing of the traumatic event in the here and now, (2) avoidance of traumatic reminders, and (3) a persistent sense of current threat. Complex post-traumatic stress disorder (CPTSD) includes the three PTSD clusters and three additional clusters that reflect disturbances in self-organization: (1) affective dysregulation, (2) negative self-concept, and (3) disturbances in relationships (Karatzias, 2018).

14:
Enter POTS

The morning was beautiful and the sun had already begun to peek behind my curtains. I reached up to take the curtain down and…

That was the last I remembered as I lay on my back, looking up at the ceiling. Everything hurt inside and I could barely move my head without feeling the wave of nausea hit. My scalp hurt and I reached up to the place that was most tender but stopped short, afraid of what I might find. Instead, I turned to look at the metal heater against the wall. A large U-shaped dent cut into the top portion—the shape of my head.

I had no idea how long I had been passed out on the floor. It made no sense to go to the doctor about this because I was just overly tired, or my anxiety had likely caught me off guard.

In addition to the head injury, I had been dealing with recurring UTI's lately, as well as spontaneous vomiting, again from stress. A sudden rapid heart rate would spontaneously occur, something I would deal with for most of my life going forward. After a time, I was diagnosed: Postural orthostatic tachycardia syndrome (POTS). This is a disorder of the autonomic nervous system involving the vagus nerve and consists of rapidly increasing heart rate while standing. It is often seen in people with autoimmune disorders, Ehlers-Danlos syndrome, and Lyme disease. But that wasn't my only issue—my jaw developed severe pain.

I had been diagnosed with temporal mandibular joint (TMJ) disorder at this time. Finally! It had been a long time suffering with TMJ pain. In addition, an X-ray showed the effects of a dislocating jaw that had agonized me for years. My jawbone was already 30% worn down by the age of 20. The TMJ and orthodontic specialist warned me that there is no jawbone replacement available and we would have to address this immediately. I had to wear a splint 24/7 while I returned to school and was scheduled to have braces put back on to correct bite, stop my jawbone from sliding out of socket, and continue to wear down. I had to have braces for a year, which meant I would have them on for my 21st birthday, unfortunately. We opted for clear braces on the top front teeth.

15:
Ski Season and a Cry For Help

"Ski season is here. Let's hit the slopes," my boyfriend said, then told me he'd be over in 30 minutes to pick me up. We were headed for the mountains and I was going to ski, even though my joints hurt and the cold altitude would only exacerbate the pain. Still, I gave it my best effort. I was slow and my joints continued to ache.

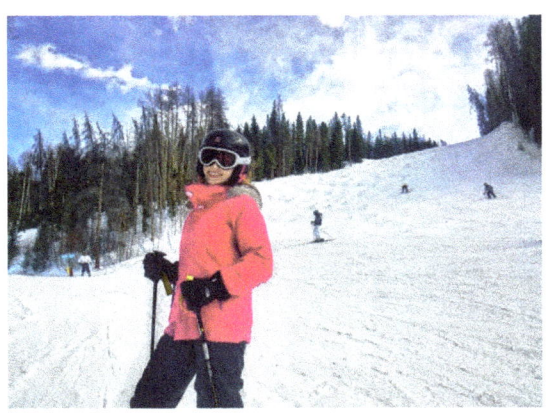

"You know, normal people make it down the hill easily in ten to fifteen minutes, tops!" he quipped.

I looked at my watch. It had been an hour since we stepped off the lift. Glancing at him, I said, "Look, I may not be the fastest up here, but I made it down. I'm really proud of myself for doing it, too."

He grunted and said, "You could try a little harder."

I paused and took in a breath of the clean, fresh mountain air. "I need to tell you something."

He gave me a look that made it clear he was in a hurry to get going again—talking wasn't his idea of a good day in snow. "What is it now?"

I swallowed and continued, "It's not entirely my fault I'm not very good at skiing, or any other sport, for that matter." I swallowed again and noticed my mouth was suddenly dry. "Look, I have Lyme disease. That's why it always takes me so long to do things, and why I'm just not as physically capable as 'normal' people. I need a pass once in a while, if I'm not performing the way you think I should."

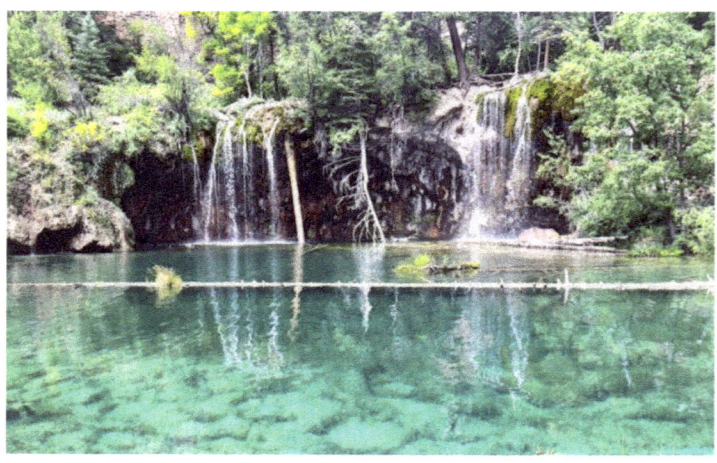

15: Ski Season and a Cry For Help

It hadn't entirely "clicked" that I was still struggling with Lyme, although I knew it was a factor. I just thought I had lasting fatigue and joint pain as a result of the disease. The symptoms never abated, even in the summertime when we would hike up to Hanging Lake, which took hours for me to accomplish. The elevation, along with joint pain and tight asthmatic breaths were a painful and difficult combination. He never understood why I was so slow, but I made it. Whatever we attempted athletically, I tried hard to participate and I accomplished that goal. I was proud. Truly, Hanging Lake was one of the most stunning places I had ever been in my life—a reward in itself.

One of the most challenging tasks undertaken at this time was in trying to find answers about my crippling anxiety. My irregular heartbeat was the most terrifying. Even without Adderall, my heart rate would beat uncontrollably fast. They call it tachycardia in the medical field—my thought was an inevitable explosion of that very organ.

Often, I would run out of my class, grabbing my chest, in fear my heart would explode. I mentioned this to my parents and my dad elected to come out to stay with me, just to keep an eye on my heart.

The usual blood work done via labs resulted in a new doctor stating, "There's nothing wrong. It's just anxiety." I was used to that type of symptom dismissal by now, but she suggested Prozac for panic attacks, which I agreed to try.

She also suggested I find a therapist.

Lyme disease patients are often dismissed as being victims of psychological illness. This happens in lieu of physical symptoms that are a normal pathophysiological course for the disease. Often, such dismissal fuels PTSD in patients, only increasing the devastation of being a victim of Lyme.

Post-traumatic stress disorder has been studied and treated successfully for years. New therapies within the cognitive behavioral therapy (CBT) realm have proven tremendously successful. As studies continue, additional causes and treatments are identified.

Unfortunately, many people who present with physical complaints may not realize their symptoms result from past traumatic experiences. In truth, the medical professionals treating these individuals also may not realize the extent of the past trauma's effect on their client's physical health and, as a result, may not correlate symptoms with history. Karatzias et al (2018) pinpoint a study conducted on the effects of complex post-traumatic stress disorder (CPTSD) and its associations

The most important correlation of CPTSD was negative cognitions about the self, characterized by a generalized negative view about the self and one's trauma symptoms; followed by attachment anxiety which is defined as involving a fear of interpersonal rejection or abandonment and/or distress if one's partner is unresponsive or unavailable; and expressive suppression, conveyed by efforts to hide, inhibit, or reduce emotional expression.

To say that I experienced symptoms based on trauma from being ill (or from previous symptoms) is an understatement. The crux of the issue lay in my history, which was not validated or considered by most medical professionals. Their focus appeared to be on mitigating the symptoms with medication. That approach often worked temporarily, but it did not address the cause. Thus, the symptoms continued which created additional symptoms with time.

15: Ski Season and a Cry For Help

My body was screaming for attention to be placed on the cause of all these related and unrelated symptoms. No one recognized the correlation. I was begging for help but was listening to what I was really saying? As a result, the trauma intensified, and I became a victim of complex post-traumatic stress disorder of the most egregious type.

Thankfully, my dad heard my cries for help. He found a psychologist who believed in mindfulness and mediation and had studied with Deepak Chopra.

16:
"It's Just Anxiety?"

"Kaitlyn, are you getting any of this?"

The therapist's words stung. I'd been with her for nearly a year—she knew me and knew how difficult all of this was for me.

"Of course," I replied.

"Well," she sighed, "it just feels like pulling teeth, trying to get you to open up every session."

That hurt my feelings and after that, I had trouble trusting her. She was judging me, like every other medical professional had done. I guess I wasn't doing things right, in her mind, and I thought I *was* confiding and opening up appropriately. This was my first experience with psych therapy. Aren't the therapists supposed to guide and take the lead in the sessions?

Things got so bad that year that my dad was forced to drive out during the second semester to help me finish my classes. It was the only way, outside of dropping out of school. He drove to campus in his car and stayed in a hotel close to my house.

Every day, I would go to where he stayed, sit there, and work on homework with him in the room, monitoring me as I cried through panic attack after panic attack, my heart racing and that familiar feeling that it would soon explode, haunting me day-in and day-out. I'm not sure I could have finished the school year without his support.

"It's just anxiety," they insisted.

"It's not anxiety," I pushed back. I didn't care that each person had the initials M. D. behind their name. "This isn't normal and it's not just stress."

It turned out to be a relapse from Lyme disease. Fortunately, the professor I approached about the symptoms and the Lyme in general, asking for an extension (and a little compassion), understood.

"I have suffered from anxiety and panic, myself, for many years," he said, smiling. "Go ahead and take your time."

My work wasn't my best quality, even with the extension, but he gave me an A- for that semester (I finished with a near 4.0 gpa that semester—something I was very proud of despite the many struggles and roadblocks faced at that time). Again, I was proud of my effort and the outcome, in spite of my health and mental health challenges.

Along with the summer came the realization that a new therapist needed to be found. She had big, curly hair and was rather shy and I felt safe with her. She taught me about the spiral of anxiety and how important it is to catch the beginning of that spiral early because, once in that spiral, it would be rather hard to stop. Often, she would take her hand and make a big spiraling motion moving upward to demonstrate a panic attack.

It made total sense to me.

Later that year, I saw a psychiatrist in Newport Beach that ended up firing me as a patient. She had prescribed Abilify for me and when I explained to her that the medication made me so exhausted that I couldn't function, she wasn't happy. It got to the point where my Lyme disease had begun to act up again, and I tried to explain that I couldn't make it to

15: "It's Just Anxiety?"

our appointment, and would she consider talking to me over the phone?

"I've even gained 30 pounds in just two months," I added, hoping she would recognize the side effects that Abilify had on my body.

"Well, that's not typical for that medication. You must not be telling the complete story because it's not possible to be that tired all the time while taking Abilify the way it's prescribed. It sounds as if you're abusing your meds."

I was confused. What a bizarre reaction from her over *my* fatigue!

"You know what? You are not the right psychiatrist for me if you cannot listen to what I'm saying and recognize problems with the medication for care that you prescribe for me! How dare you call me a liar!" I hung up the phone and quickly found a different psychiatrist to monitor my meds.

As soon as I came off the Abilify, the weight dropped off. Apparently, my personality improved as well—I wasn't flat and lethargic any longer, but that meant the apprehension and panic would return. Anxiety was something I couldn't escape, it seemed.

17:
Not the guy

It was time to get as mentally strong as I could in preparation for my senior year, the fall of 2014. Thankfully, I no longer had to live in the moldy house and elected, instead, to move into a newer, healthier townhouse. My room was the largest with a skylight and sizeable window that overlooked an immense, beautiful tree. I had renewed hope that this coming year would be better. Classes started and I turned 21 in that same season. We celebrated with dinner, dancing, and a traditional kiss of the buffalo (a tradition at Boulder). Things definitely looked brighter!

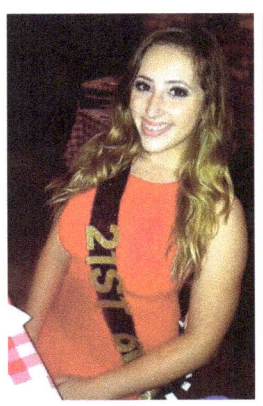
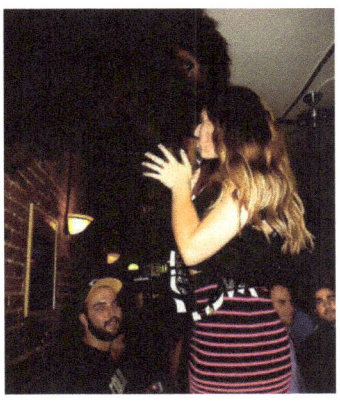

At first I did okay with alcohol—until I didn't. I began to have extreme detox reactions to alcohol even in small amounts. One night specifically I had one to two drinks and vomited all day the next day, shaking and in agony. Lyme disease patients can have adverse reactions to alcohol because it triggers a severe Herxheimer reaction.

And then, my boyfriend turned the tables… again.

"I think it's best we end this," he announced out of the blue.

I tore off my "Love" necklace and ended up breaking the clasp. The tears wouldn't stop, and I found myself begging for another chance. This was his decision. I knew I hadn't done anything wrong, but still, the need to have him in my life propelled me to believe I wasn't strong enough without him.

I mean, that's love, isn't it?

There was nowhere to go except to my other friends, many of whom were male. So, I leaned on them for support. This made him jealous. In one of my therapy sessions, I mentioned my boyfriend and his inability to tolerate my illness, or anything else.

"Why don't you bring him in on our next session. That way, I can get to know him a little bit, possibly help you both."

Arrangements were made and he agreed to accompany me to the next session. Once we arrived, he declined to get out of the car. He cried and refused to even shake her hand or say "Hi." When I walked into the therapist's office and explained what was happening outside in the car, she simply shook her head and said, "Kaitlyn, this is not the guy for you."

I dropped my eyes. I knew she was right.

"I mean," she continued, "if he isn't willing to do what is asked of him, to help you feel supported, he's not the right one."

I said nothing in response. She was right.

18:
My Grandma, Uncle, and a Betta Fish

Late October arrived and the shift in the weather matched my mood—cool, breezy, and colorful. Mom came in town for a visit and we had a fun day driving around sight-seeing together. At dinner, the Christmas holidays came up and my anticipation increased at the thought of family times during the Christmas season.

"Maybe we can see grandma." I said. "Christmas is so much fun with her, with everyone together…"

My mom shook her head. "Something's happened."

The look in my mother's eyes chased away my appetite. I could only ask, "What?" afraid of the answer.

"She died. Grandma died, honey."

My mouth went dry and my eyes filled with tears. I could no longer stay in the restaurant and ran to the car desperate to escape the truth. Mom grabbed food boxes and followed me out then sat quietly as I cried and cried.

Italian food never tasted the same after that.

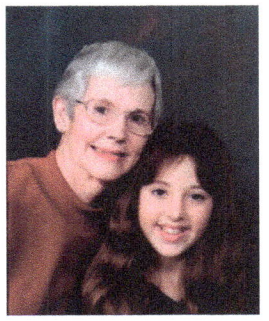

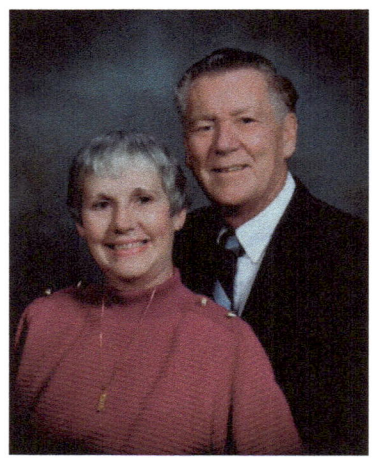
Grandma Maona and Grandpa Orville

Halloween rolled around about the same time we prepared for grandma's funeral. I thought dressing in coordinated costumes might ease some of the pain from losing her—maybe even bring a little "fun" into a bleak month. My boyfriend agreed and when Halloween night finally arrived, I did my best to get ready, ready to go out and celebrate in style.

"You're taking too long. This is ridiculous!" he snapped. "We'll miss everything at this pace."

"I'm doing my best."

He shook his head and began to pace. "It's not just that. You're re-kindling old flames. I know it."

I was flabbergasted. His intolerance for my inability to keep up to his expectations was unbelievable. Add to that, the accusation he leveled at me and I had no words. The fight that ensued was brutal. My effort to explain how my body was slowing down meant nothing to him. Defensiveness didn't either, in fact, it infuriated him further. We walked home in silence that night. I knew it was over.

18: My Grandma, Uncle, and a Betta Fish

Grandma's funeral was held in Missouri. Sadly, my uncle did not look well and collapsed carrying the casket at the funeral. Thankfully, he was alright and returned to the house where he found me arguing over the phone with my boyfriend—the whole thing started over a joke I made about his birthday party. I guess he didn't think it was funny. Unfortunately, I missed saying goodbye to my uncle because of this fight. It was the last opportunity I would be given to say anything to my uncle… thanks to a fight.

I flew home to a huge final project for one of my classes. My boyfriend wanted to see me as soon as I arrived and wouldn't take "no" for an answer when I tried to explain the pressure I was under to finish this project for school.

"I'll be there in a minute," he announced.

"No!" I said and locked the doors.

Distractions meant that I wouldn't finish and I couldn't risk it, given the time I had just spent for grandma's funeral.

"Just open the door," he said, peeking through the glass window. My roommate unlocked the door and let him in. Taking the stairs two at a time, he pushed through the defective lock on my bedroom door.

"It's really over this time. I'm breaking up with you."

It was too much for me—his moody demands and the burdens of school. "Okay, then get the f*ck out."

"Don't you at least want to know why?"

"Not really," I said glancing down at the papers spread all over my desk. By now, it was obvious to me that anyone who disregards a request for privacy, who breaks up the day after a funeral, and who shows no tolerance or respect toward me is not a good person… not the person I want in my life. "You sneak into my house after I asked you to *not* come over and your lack of tolerance for anything that doesn't fit your expectations shows your true colors. I don't like the person you are. Now, get out!"

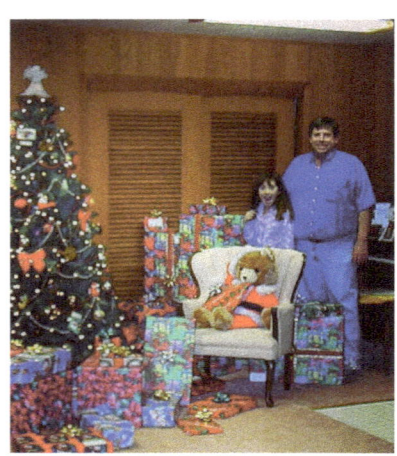

He left.

The relief that followed was short-lived. That same week, my favorite pet betta fish died—I had planned to take him home with me. I also found out that my uncle (the uncle to whom I never said "goodbye") died, as well.

He was only 57.

My heart was broken.

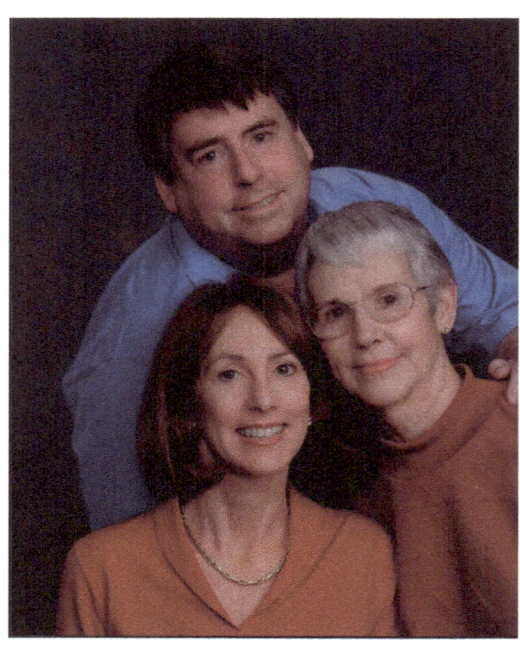

My uncle Gary

19:
Loss

Loss is one of the highest ranked events on the list of life-stressors. Multiple loss is devastating. I had suffered the latter and was not able to finish my project, as a result. I walked down for class the next morning and met two of my roommates, carrying huge packets in hand.

"What have you got there?" I asked.

The response was not one I was prepared to hear. "Our final projects."

I had completely forgotten about the project for my primate class and had failed the last exam I'd taken after grandma's death. There was no chance now of passing the class.

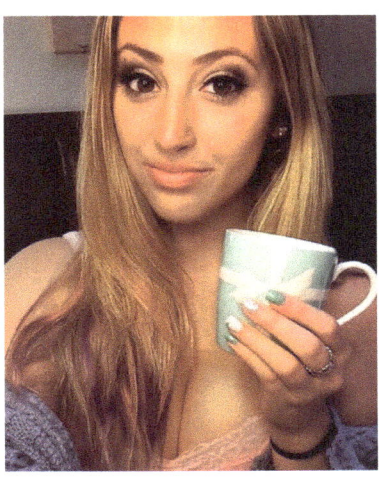

I went blonde my senior year after my breakup and double loss. The stress of the situation on campus had become too much, and I began to develop stress incontinence of my bladder. One day, while getting ready to go to class, I rushed out the door, in a hurry, apparently unaware that I had to urinate. I didn't feel like I had to urinate… until I did—a full bladder's worth. I peed my pants and was so confused and soiled that I couldn't make it to class.

"Something must be wrong," I said to the doctor in follow up to my embarrassing incontinent experience that day.

"Well, do you have more than three children?" she asked, keeping an eye on my chart in her lap.

"No! No children."

"Hmmm," she glanced up at me briefly. "This is really very rare for someone without children. You know, stress can worsen this condition."

Well, that made sense. I definitely had stress. School wasn't working out and I had few options.

The next call I made was to my parents. "I think I need to withdraw from school," was all I said. It was enough.

There was one last hope to salvage this semester. So, I contacted my counselor and asked for advice. She advised about the withdrawal process due to the family death.

"That's good to know, but honestly, I think my Lyme disease is coming back. I mean, it's not like me to fail tests and forget completely about projects. I'm a good student, really."

"I can see that," she said. "And truly I understand your situation. My mother also had Lyme disease, and so I recognize how devastating that illness can be."

My relief must have shown on my face because she smiled at me. "I am going to make a recommendation that may be difficult for you to hear, Kaitlyn. You should seriously consider withdrawing from all of your classes, including the ones you feel confident you are doing well in. It's the only way to get some money back from this semester."

"But… I…"

19: Loss

"I also recommend you take some time off and get some rest. Get better physically and mentally so that you can start fresh when you decide to return."

My therapist agreed with her. And so, I withdrew from the school one week before finals in the first semester of my senior year. All of the sudden stress, in combination with the inability to regulate my nervous system and emotions, led to a horrific Lyme disease relapse—worse than I had ever experienced before.

20:
Fear for My safety

Sleep overtook my time after I had withdrawn from school. I seemed to need it, more than before, anyway. My memory was also affected, and not for the better. I couldn't remember anything—whether I had handed my card to a barista to pay or not, and I would have to ask. It was very uncomfortable.

California seemed like the perfect place to recover, and so I went home for winter break and hung out with my friends. I saw my California therapist while there in hopes that she could help me with the healing process.

It was then that I received anti-Semitic threats from someone who claimed to go to school with me. They threatened with comments such as, "Just wait until you get back to campus." I wasn't sure what that meant for me but I knew I didn't want to find out.

I was called a "Jewish piece of trash."

Personal information was shared about me that included information about my father's side of the family, who were all Jewish. This was a fact I usually kept private, except to my close family and friends.

I reported it to the police and they told me I would need to have a police escort from class to class if I chose to go back to Colorado. On top of everything else, I now would now have to worry about my physical safety on campus.

I tried to return and re-enrolled in classes, in spite of the therapists' and counselors' advice. I made it a full week before withdrawing again, just before the drop deadline.

Suddenly, I began to have ideas of how to create things and started ordering Amazon packages for myself. This may have been the beginning of manic behavior.

I didn't feel particularly safe physically on campus and wasn't ready to return to school, just yet. My parents had driven with all of our pets to Missouri. So, I decided I would join them for a while in an attempt to heal. I attempted a "goodbye" to my ex-boyfriend because I was sure it could be the last time I would ever see him again.

He never looked me in the eye. Obviously, things didn't go well. So, I got on the plane and left. It was the last time I ever saw him.

21:
Music and the Influencer Era

I had missed my flight. It wasn't my fault, really. I was just so tired.

There was no energy to clean my room or pack or move my car to the spot it would need to stay put for the semester.

I cried a lot.

I would have to reschedule the flight to Missouri, rest, and try again.

My parents ordered a car to have me taken to the airport so that the missed-flight event wouldn't recur. During the ride, my palms were clammy and my body broke out into a full sweat. Thankfully, there was air-conditioning in the vehicle—it seemed to help enough to keep my wits together enough to leave.

When I arrived in Missouri, I was greeted by my mom's new red teacup poodle puppy. He was pure joy!

While there, I sang a little bit and soon realized I wanted to focus on music for a bit. It was time to take a break from school. So, I sang, traveled, and took photos of different places in Missouri.

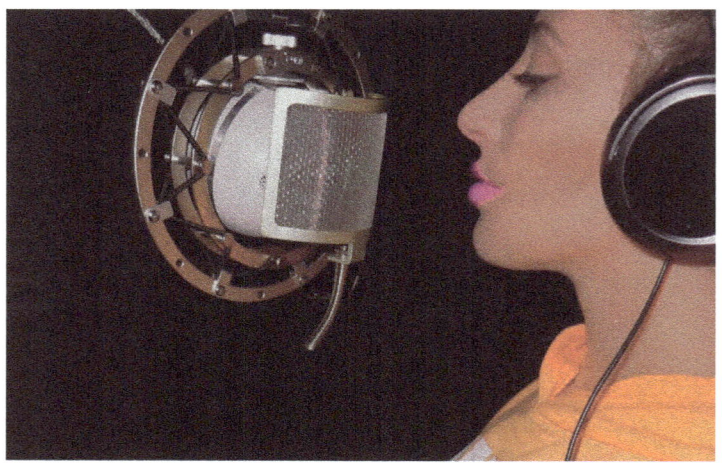

During this same trip, my dad visited some property located in deep brush. He returned covered in large ticks. One was stuck in his armpit. I improperly pulled it out with a pair of tweezers. He ended up in the ER to have the rest of the embedded tick removed, and I immediately grew concerned, asking him to query about the possibility of Doxycycline for treatment. The ER doctor said no, suggesting that the large ticks are not usually Lyme carriers. In his opinion, it is the small ticks (like the one we found on my leg) that are prone to carry Lyme. I still think it would have been in his best interest to insist on receiving a round of antibiotics, but he ended up being fine and without symptoms.

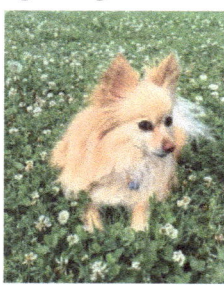

Another time, I found a large, swollen grey tick behind my Pomeranian-Chihuahua's ear. This occurred from Coco's exploring our back yard in Missouri. I removed it and she also seemed to be okay after this, as well. The Lyme disease vaccine in dogs is not safe and can actually cause more adverse symptoms than

21: Music and the Influencer Era

help (some believe it can actually transfer Lyme to the dog), so we elected to wait for signs of developing symptoms. Luckily, that wasn't her fate.

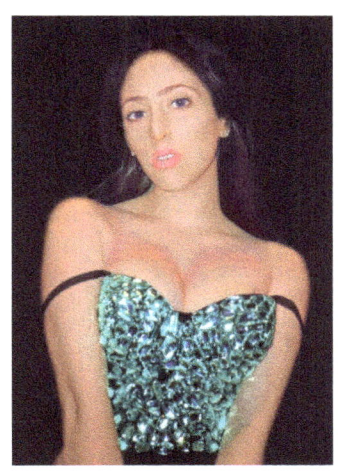

I stayed in Missouri for the entirety of the semester, and then returned when my lease was up, mainly to get my stuff, drive my car and bring my new fish back with me to California. Once settled again, I returned to voice lessons and started doing open mics.

On the internet, I started to post my singing, fashion, and photography regularly, specifically onto Instagram. There, I built up a following.

Collaboration offers came in for different companies, which let me take photos with their products to post to my Instagram account. I started singing in public during this time but had trouble memorizing the lyrics and would get the familiar, horrible racing heart and panic attacks on performance day.

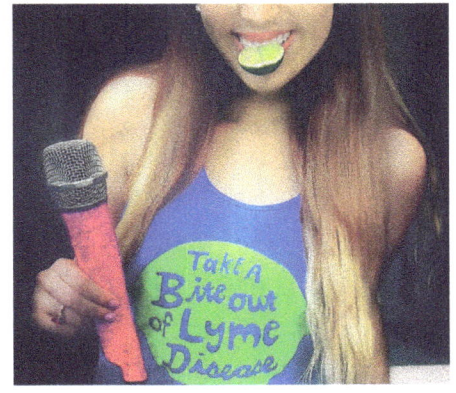

Like clockwork, I began to get worse every Wednesday. My voice instructor suggested it might be stage-fright or anxiety. I knew it was more than that. I would be able to stand during the entire set, print out or use an iPad for the lyrics, then power through the panic attacks. Occasionally, the panic attack was so bad that I'd raise the white flag and be forced to cancel.

Now and then, I dated a few people but… nothing really stuck.

My kidney and bladder issues worsened. Recurring bladder infections progressed into the kidneys and caused tremendous back pain and vomiting. This alone made it impossible to go on a date, let alone go out to dinner. Hives, rashes, redness, and dermatographic urticaria (skin writing) all followed. I could scratch a smiley face into my arm with my fingernail and it would stay there for long periods of time. The whole thing was time-consuming! Hours every morning were spent in an allergist's office with each infection after taking antibiotics, just to make sure I wasn't going to go into anaphylactic shock. The whole process was degrading and very discouraging.

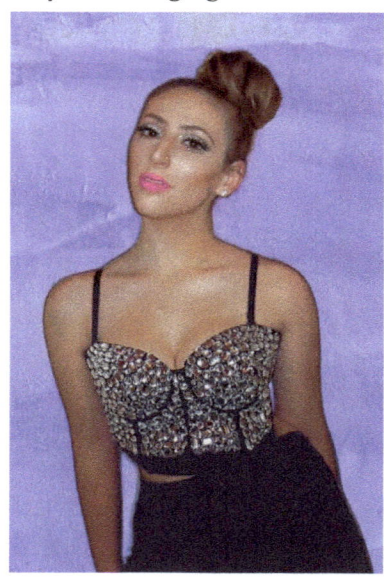

To lessen the angst, I took up horseback riding again. The lessons included jumping small fences and care for my horse afterward. This routine threw me back into bed for two days afterward, but I loved it so much that I chose to ignore the repercussions and continued the lessons. Given my limited strength, I didn't have the energy to cook and relied, instead, on Starbucks and/or takeout. I physically looked great and

21: Music and the Influencer Era

was in the best shape of my life at this time. There was much to be thankful for, which was great for the Instagram content.

I had been managing like this until one day, I couldn't. I developed severe vomiting and was so weak I couldn't sit upright. Still, in that weakened condition, I was alert enough one night to hear drilling coming from my driveway, outside my window. The next day, I discovered thieves had stolen the metal roof runners off of my car.

The sickness and stress sent me to the doctor the next day. He examined me and looked concerned. "You're yellow."

"I am? What does that mean?" I asked, equally concerned.

"What other symptoms are you experiencing?"

I thought for a minute then gushed, "Severe fatigue, vomiting so bad that I can't even keep water down, and I'm so lethargic that I missed the thieves stealing pieces off of my car."

He didn't seem to notice the last of my concerns and simply replied, "I think you might have Hepatitis A from contaminated food or water." He never followed up with a blood test, but later tests were positive for Hepatitis A antibodies. I believe his observations and resulting diagnosis were correct. "Go home, rest, hydrate and give it time. It will go away on its own."

At this point, I knew I needed to come clean with my parents and not sugar-coat my symptoms and what was really going on with my body. The search began for information about long-term or chronic Lyme symptoms. Following other Lyme patients on social media and chatting with some of them became a priority. Many of us had the same symptoms.

Whenever I tried to explain to my parents what I had discovered, at first they reacted with distrust, stating emphatically that I was "listening to other people and getting brainwashed in the process." This was extremely hurtful. It took them coming home to see how sick I really was before they understood.

22:
Lyme Literacy

"Certainly, there are Lyme-literate medical professionals somewhere!" I stated aloud to no one in particular.

The search commenced and I soon discovered that additional information had been added into the 2016 guidelines for "What to do if you think you have Lyme disease," especially chronic Lyme disease.

The physician generator became a very useful tool in which to locate doctors in the area, all the way up to Washington State. Three doctors were suggested by the generator, all located in my area. After a bit of vetting, I picked the one I thought was the best fit. Another girl in my area appeared on Instagram. She also had Lyme and asked if I could go to brunch with her, to meet and hopefully give her some guidance.

I agreed and we met that week. She told me that she had used the same doctor I had picked from the list and mentioned, "That doctor saved my life."

Right then and there, I decided that this would be my doctor.

Lyme Pivot. It's a thing.

The Center for Disease Control (CDC) pivots. A timeline of when the CDC used to accept chronic Lyme in began in 1990. They then pivoted to 2000 for political reasons, stating that chronic Lyme doesn't exist. Currently, their explanation of PTLDS remains—a pivot.

In truth, the CDC has a complicated relationship with "Chronic Lyme disease." Chronic is the debated word. It was accepted in 1990 as a legitimate diagnosis. In 2000, they pivoted, stating it's not accepted and not true. After long covid, they were pressured into accepting that some of the long term symptoms were real and decided to edit their position, not stating that some patients do, in fact, have long term symptoms. This happened in December of 2023.

23:
Tests, Tests, and More Tests

The day before Halloween in 2016, I met with the LLMD in Orange County and received multiple diagnoses in the process. I'm not sure whether that made me feel better or worse. One specific diagnosis, Mast Cell Activation Syndrome (MCAS), was new—I had never heard of such an illness. But this diagnosis finally explained the strange rashes and hives, especially when given antibiotics.

The proof was in the research. Fortunately, this doctor had done hers and the results spelled out my story very clearly.

Lyme disease, the most prevalent tick-associated disease in the United States, is a chronic inflammatory disorder caused by spirochetes of *Borrelia burgdorferi* sensu lato (14). Early symptoms of infection include fatigue, joint and muscle pain, and, in approximately 60% of cases, the characteristic erythema migrans lesion. If not treated, secondary pathological symptoms may manifest as arthritis, carditis, and neurologic disorders (Talkington et al, 1999).

According to the study above, mast cells activated by spirochetes probably contribute to subsequent immune and/

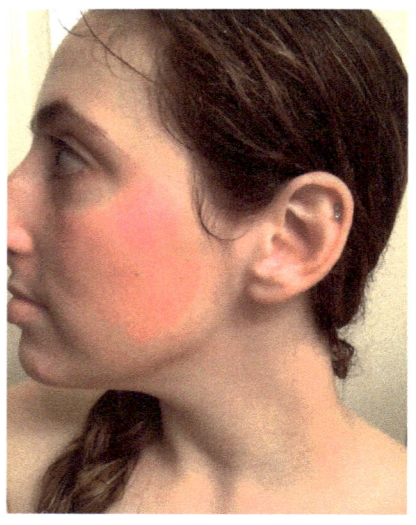

or inflammatory events. This seemed to be my course. As a result, my new physician (an integrative medical doctor and Lyme-literate medical doctor) decided to test me for what felt like every illness and syndrome known to mankind.

The blood tests had to be broken up into two different days. The first day alone was 15-20 vials of blood, during which I lost my vision, thought I would pass out, and had to lay down.

This physician continued to delve into possibilities for causes and became suspicious of Ehlers Danlos Syndrome. When I explained my history of Lyme disease, she started me on saline IVs first and eventually IV glutathione to detox my system. On occasion, the hives would surface from the saline alone, speaking volumes about how triggered my system was.

My blood tests came back with two different types of immunodeficiency: Primary (low IgG) and secondary (low IgA), along with and hyper IgE syndrome. Finally, someone found the answers as to why I got sick every year. Unfortunately, until then, no one had even thought to test my immune system, and of course, I wasn't aware these tests existed until this physician's evaluation.

My Lyme disease test came back negative. I didn't have the knowledge at this time to ask to look for specifics details or to look for any positive bands. It is my belief that the physician only tested me for American Lyme disease, but I cannot be

23: Tests, Tests, and More Tests

sure of it. Had she had tested for European Lyme disease; the answers may have surfaced sooner. At least the CDC test was negative on this round of this testing, but is well-known, being CDC-negative does not mean one doesn't have Lyme disease.

One would think that whatever the CDC recommends is trustworthy or that the tests conducted by them are completely accurate—but that's not always the case, according to the experts at IGeneX Inc. (2024). Historically, only two main tests were available: The Western Blot test and the ELISA. More recent assay variations have allowed for a broader scope of testing and diagnoses for Lyme disease. Sadly, even with a greater variety of testing to utilize for diagnosis purposes, not all medical professionals are aware of the serious complexities or symptomatology of Lyme disease. As the experts at IGeneX Inc., (2024) state, "...finding a Lyme-literate medical doctor (LLMD) can make a world of difference. Lyme disease is the most frequently misdiagnosed tick-borne disease. Going to a doctor that knows what symptoms to look for at different stages and what your testing options are can help you get an accurate diagnosis and suitable treatment"—a crucial step to identifying and improving Lyme disease's effects.

Once a diagnosis is obtained, it becomes vital to recognize the significance that inflammation plays in the pathogenesis of the disease. Caused by the spirochete, *Borrelia burgdorferi*, the host defense is affected, with glutathione (GSH) metabolism most affected (Kerstholt et al (2018). These authors continue to discuss the "modulating GSH metabolism significantly affects cytokine production, possibly through glutathionylation. We provide evidence that GSH metabolism is altered in patients with erythema migrans (EM)" the rash commonly seen with Lyme disease, "and that these alterations might persist for months after the initial infection" if left untreated, identified as inflammatory responses in the joints, heart, and/or nervous system. The urgency to identify the source of these symptoms is without question. Further research and utilization of appropriate testing will support physician recognition of this devastating disease and hopefully, allow for an earlier treatment plan of care for their Lyme disease patients.

24:
A New Friend and an LLMD

I made a new best friend who also suffered with Lyme disease. This happened through Instagram. She had tried numerous treatments and was able to guide me through my own process.

The treatment began slowly. My LLMD started me on an IV drip of saline and glutathione. In 2016, that was the best treatment for what was assumed my problem that included mast cell activation syndrome (MCAS). The treatment included B12 and a cocktail of other medications.

"I think it's helping," I said one day.

"Great!" came the response. "I still want to explore other possibilities, like Ehlers Danlos that we talked about." I knew in my gut that this was Lyme but I stayed with her and trusted the process. "Let's get you approved for something called IVIG. It works to boost an inadequate immune system. But I must give a little warning here," she paused to look at me and my family a little more sternly, "it's going to be a tough road."

I swallowed and felt my stomach lurch. Dad must have felt the same because he leaned forward in his chair and asked her, "What do you mean by tough?"

"Well, you'll have to really fight the insurance company to approve this. But more than that, if we leave this untreated, whatever has affected Kaitlyn will only get much worse."

No one said anything for a while.

"During the treatment phase?" I finally asked.

The doctor smiled. "I'm afraid so. The treatment will take a couple of years to complete, two to be exact, and you will likely feel worse before you start to feel better."

I didn't want to believe her at first, this couldn't be the best course of action. But I trusted her and she had been correct about everything thus far. I decided to continue with her suggestions and tried to prepare myself for what lay ahead. Again, she was dead-on with these predictions. Things were about to get a lot worse.

Insurance companies aren't always the first to get on board with medication treatment options for rare diseases. And while Lyme isn't necessarily rare, it still falls into that grey area for

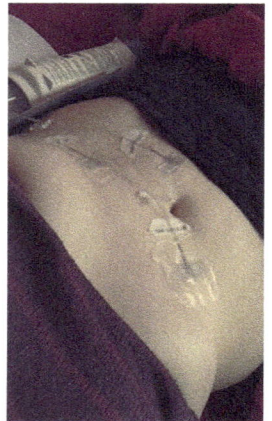

pharmacy support. Sadly, it would take until February 3, 2018, to get IVIG approved. My insurance company let me suffer with a weakened immune system for years.

Lyme disease, even with extensive antibiotic treatment, can still lead to long-term symptomatology and the now-recognized Lyme disease syndrome. Fortunately, studies have shown effective treatments available that include glutathione (GSH).

24: A New Friend and an LLMD

Pathway analysis indicated that glutathione (GSH) metabolism was the pathway most significantly affected by *Bb*. Lyme disease, caused by *Borrelia burgdorferi* (*Bb*) *sensu lato*, is the most common vector-borne disease in the Northern hemisphere, transmitted by ticks. Lyme disease most often presents locally with a migrating skin rash called erythema migrans (EM) but, if left untreated, can give rise to inflammatory complications in the joints, heart, or nervous system (Kerstholt et al, 2018).

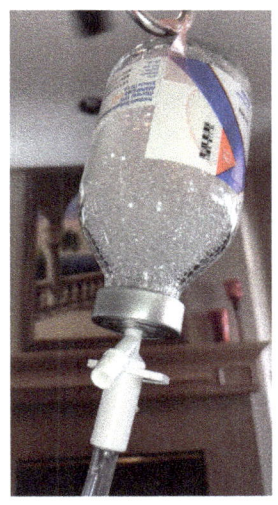

In a nutshell, Borrelia burgdorferi (Bb) is a very forceful initiator of cytokines that lead to an inflammatory response found in Lyme disease, specifically inflammation that advances to arthritis. Though still under study, there is conclusive evidence that glutathione provides positive treatment results, particularly when combined with B12.

It worked for me to help me detox and be prepared for stronger treatment. Interestingly, my doctor wanted to look deeper into the possibility of mold and heavy metals. I did tests for both. Nothing remarkable was discovered with the mold levels—basically, they were okay. I tested slightly higher for Gadolinium, but that finding wasn't one she too concerned about.

The result: It wasn't mold, it wasn't heavy metal exposure causing my issues.

I started to get weaker and more fatigued. Now that I knew my immunity was compromised, I was afraid of getting sick and began to isolate a little more. The year was 2017, and Morgellons entered my life. Soon after, I received my clinical Lyme diagnosis.

25:
There's Something Inside of Me

"What is that?"

It swirled and twisted as the water gradually changed colors—a deathly ashen pastiness that couldn't be good. "Water isn't supposed to look like that. And what is that swimming around in the tub with me?

I glanced down, checking to make sure I could still see my legs. The skin poised just above the surface was covered in lesions. I reached up to push strands of hair off of my face and discovered handfuls full of long strands in clumps between my fingers.

A bath was meant to be soothing, peaceful, cleansing but the water had turned grey and was filled with hoary fibers, swirling in strange patterns as the water moved in strange ways. I believed these fibers had come out of my lesions.

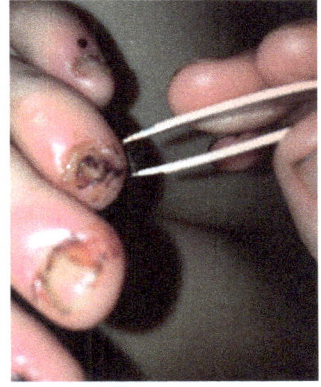

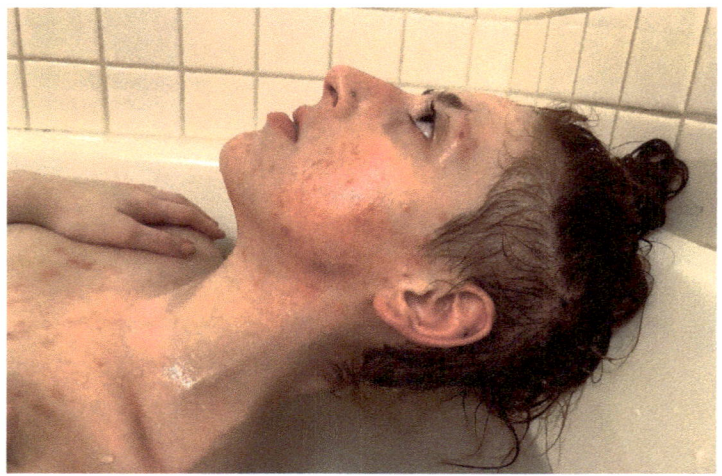

I mentioned this to my doctor, who examined my lesions and suggested I be tested for parasites. I was not allowed back into the Lyme doctor's office until I received negative tests for parasites.

So, I went back to the ER and the doctors there also examined my lesions, then suggested I was somehow creating the lesions that ran up and down my back, using tools, and then intentionally sticking fibers into my skin.

Their answer was a printed list of psychiatrists.

A huge part of my life included the creation of content 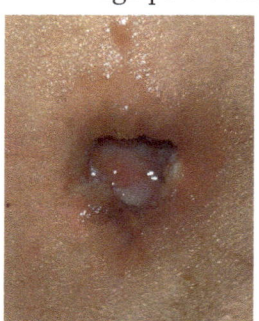 for Instagram at this time. The last thing I wanted to do was harm myself, especially my skin, particularly on my face that had recently broken out into huge, deep lesions across my forehead and cheekbones. The lesions covered my legs, ran up and down my spine, bespeckled my face, and peppered my arms.

25: There's Something Inside of Me

My skin would randomly start bleeding and I'd spit out or bleed cups worth of blood. My doctor diagnosed me with necrosis and said it could be part of the process. Fluid poured out and one hole to my hip tore 5 inches into my skin and tissue. Something that looked like gravel came out of the hole. I was afraid of the ER at this point because they were so dismissive and refused to go even though I could stick my finger all the way in my skin to my hip. I had an IVIG nurse that happened to specialize in wound care who monitored the wound, flushed it with saline, and packed the hole until it healed.

My doctor suggested an infectious disease doctor to test for parasites, so I brought samples to a hospital lab. Not long afterward, the doctor called and stated, "Everything came back negative for parasites. You have something called Morgellons Disease. You have Lyme disease and now we know how to treat it."

The plan of care included a cocktail combination IV therapy of Doxycycline, Daptomycin, and Rifampin. I was given a central line, placed in my chest because the veins in my arm were starting to develop scar tissue (likely, from years of intravenous infusions). I elected to go with a Hickman catheter. Once stem cell therapy was ready, safe, and available to the public, we would follow up with this intervention to repair the damage that Lyme had done to my body and brain.

Many doctors consider this skin disorder a "delusional parasitosis" or "delusional infestation," to include "delusional filament fibers," suggesting the fibers are introduced by the victim. At least, that's what Middelveen et al (2015) claim physicians typically state.

Research and testing have shown that the fictitious fibers result from keratinocytes and fibroblasts in the skin, resulting from a disease called, Morgellons that is contracted from Lyme disease. In addition to the skin disorders (filaments and rashes), musculoskeletal and neurocognitive symptoms are noted, brought about from Lyme disease and a tick bite.

Morgellons disease is recognized as being caused by the spirochete, *Borrelia burgdorferi*. Physicians would do well to get on board with the extensive evidence supporting Morgellons disease related to Lyme disease.

Lyme borreliosis is a systemic infection that is commonly associated with dermatological manifestations. Given that most [Morgellons disease (MD)] patients are serologically reactive to [*Borrelia burgdorferi* (Bb)] antigens, the presence of Lyme spirochetes in MD dermatological lesions is predictable and supports an etiologic role of the spirochetal disease (Middelveen et al (2015).

Lyme disease and its symptomatology are real and the symptoms associated with Morgellons disease are likewise real. The somatic illnesses associated with Lyme need to be acknowledged and treated appropriately by healthcare professionals and *not* dismissed as a psychosomatic issue.

26:
Not the Antidote

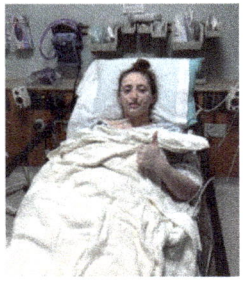

IVIG was the treatment of the day and I was one of its recipients. Sadly, the treatment only seemed to worsen my symptoms, as well as the inflammation in my brain. After a particularly bad reaction one day, we decided to stop. When the doctor considered I was strong enough, we began IV antibiotics. It had been nearly two years of sitting in bed and I began to grow delusional and paranoid. It began with planes flying over my house—I *knew* they were watching me.

27:
Out of Control

The rage was uncontrollable. I lost it with friends, family, even boyfriends any time someone disagreed or disappointed me.

"I can't control it!" was my response when questioned about why I was so angry. Their answer was to walk away. I lost most of my friends during this time period. Some due to my behavior and others seemed to just lose interest because I couldn't go out anymore.

"I can't handle this anymore, Kaitlyn." My best friend, still living in Colorado, sent over text.

"Not my fault. It's just how you've been pulling away! I need you to care."

"I'm done," she said.

I had just lost my best friend from college and it was due to one of these outbursts, although I couldn't control myself. I tried to work through it further but she had blocked me on every platform.

This was heartbreaking.

"What's going on with you?" It was an attempt by my ex to contact me. His newest relationship with a high school girlfriend didn't seem to deter his efforts.

"Leave me alone!" My response was punitive and final.

I continued with the IV antibiotics that caused an excruciating Herxheimer reaction. The only relief came as I would lay in an Epsom salt bath, still writhing in pain and often praying to either heal or not wake up the next morning. It was a dark time, but I couldn't see a way out nor a future where healing would be an outlook. Nothing seemed to help, especially during the antibiotic infusions when large red streaks appeared on my abdomen and hips. Added to the problem, I had not yet gained weight.

This likely was a sign of Bartonella.

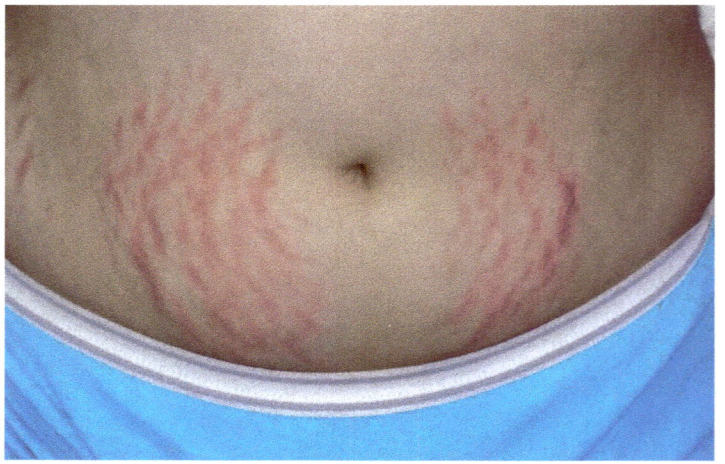

Lyme rage is more common than most people realize. The symptoms are often described as uncontrolled anger that rises out of nowhere, uncontrollable, and debilitating. One description includes experiencing "many forms of anger in the two decades I've been sick with Lyme. Anger, when no one could diagnose me with anything other than 'stress' or 'being run down.' Anger, when people told me the symptoms might all be in my head" (*Anger & Lyme disease: What to know*, 2017). Frustration always follows as a default diagnosis of "crazy" or psychological/mental illness rubber-stamps the individual with Lyme-rage, leading to medical misdiagnosis of the root cause of the rage problem.

So critical is the urgency to recognize Lyme anger in patients who carry Lyme disease or have a history of tick bites. To those who suffer from Lyme rage, I would encourage self-advocacy for additional testing to seek a "root cause" for the rage. Employ the help of a trusted LLMD.

28:
Back Again

Multiple emergency department visits followed during this time. One time, I presented with an episode in which I couldn't walk, twisting in agony. Half of my face had dropped and there was concern that I had suffered a stroke or was a victim of severe Bell's palsy. Perhaps I'd thrown a clot from the Groshong tissue that apparently had clotted my Hickman catheter (the medical staff pulled it soon after). No one followed up or answered questions about exactly what had happened.

On another presentation to the ER, my heart raced, like a freight train, and my brain felt swollen. I was told that I was "drug seeking" by asking for an IV—something that I normally would have been able to successfully request from a doctor or mobile IV clinic, if it had been standard business hours.

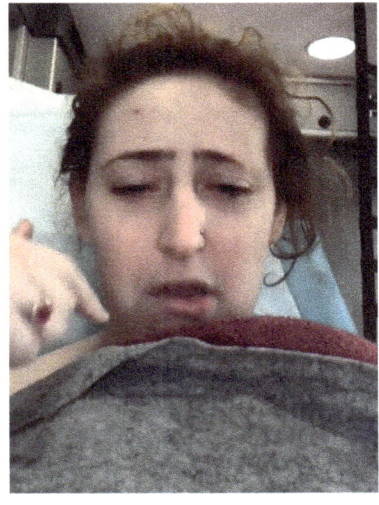

Another incident gifted me with an antibiotic-resistant "superbug" discovered in my bladder. Of course, treating that required an additional, specific antibiotic. Following that, a fourth incident left me feeling horrible, gaslit, dismissed to home. The medical team discovered their error and called back that evening with information about a very serious, life-threatening infection (sepsis) that was the cause of my symptoms.

The outcome of those events: A different hospital that immediately hospitalized and monitored my sepsis, admitting me overnight for the first time in my life.

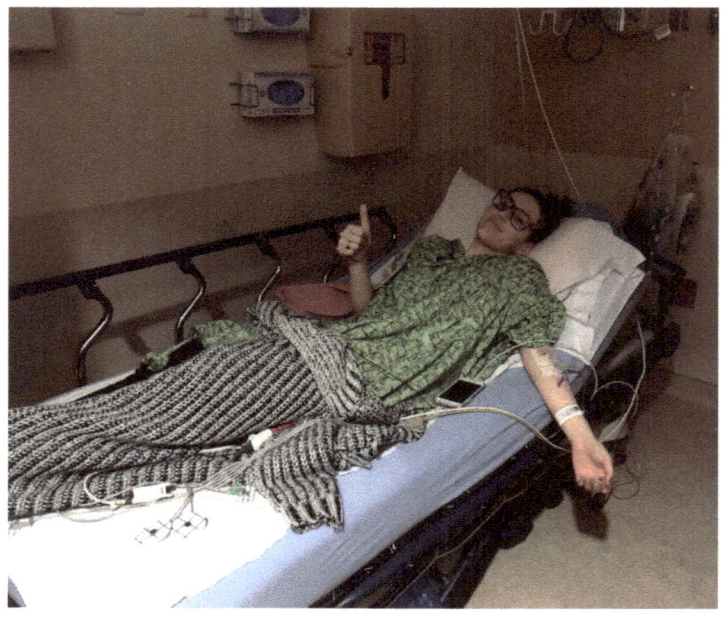

I was placed on steroids to prevent any rejection of the treatments given. My abdomen swelled and my face ballooned, along with my weight that climbed to 200 pounds in a very short amount of time. Half of my head was completely bald at

28: Back Again

this point, and the small amount of hair I had left I tied into a tiny bun on top my head.

Accompanying the physical swelling, the delusions amplified. Sadly, my beloved horse passed away, as well, from an unexpected intestinal rupture. This loosened my grip on reality until it severed completely. A running monologue of celebrity voices sounded telepathically in my head, all talking directly to me. They told me all of their secrets and that I too would be a big star one day. I believed that every song and video on Instagram mocked me or somehow was about me. I placed tape over my phone's camera because knew I was being watched.

My new best friend would sit with me, listening to me over the phone, in an attempt to comfort and help me calm down. She had also experienced mental health issues from Lyme and understood what was going on.

I was manic. I decided to purchase a horse—online and with a credit card.

After I lost my childhood horse, I prayed, asking for her to come back to me as a baby foal—one that looked similar but with stronger legs and feet. The name *Chantilly* came to me in prayer (or perhaps delusion). The first horse had Chantilly lace markings on her legs. So, it made perfect sense that my next horse's name would be Chantilly.

This began an internet search for an appaloosa filly. Surprisingly, I found an American Sugarbush Harlequin Draft horse (founded with appaloosa lines) online that was named *Chantilly* already (registered name *Heiress Apparent*). Added to my amazement, she looked very similar to the horse I had lost.

Synchronicity? Perhaps.

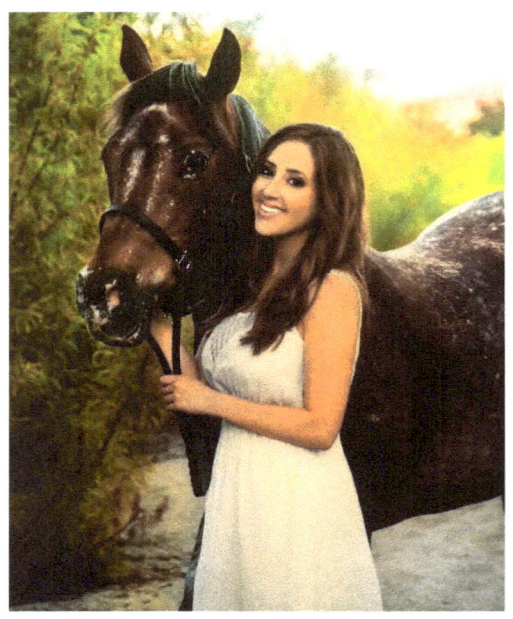

Quest Go Fancy

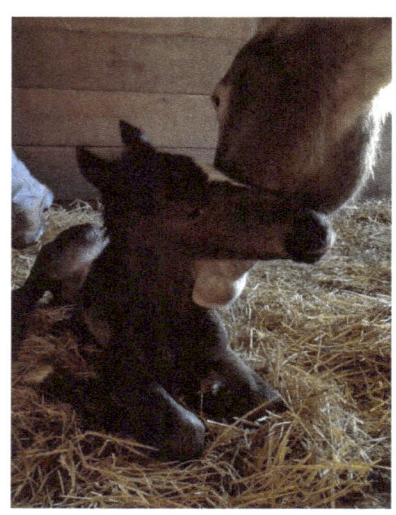

This occurred just two months before I was sent to the psych ward. Obviously, the purchase was not a well thought-out plan for many reasons

SIDE NOTE: It was the first post on Facebook —Chantilly's birth announcement that said:
She's here! Our first foal of the year! A dark bay Sugarbush filly with spots over her hips! She is FANCY!

28: Back Again

The ad went up the day my Fancy passed away —10/04/19.

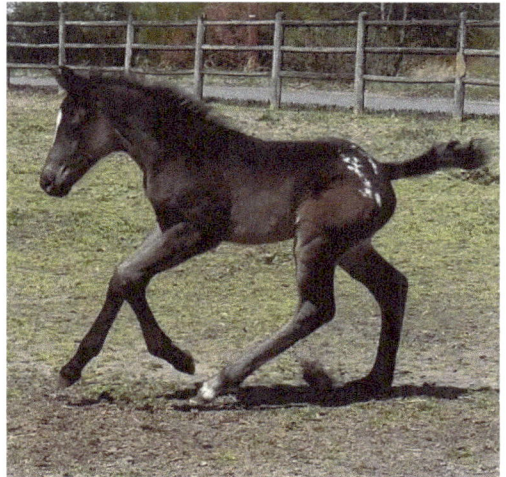

Photo credit to Trinity Appaloosa Farm

Disorder: The Great Educator

"Bipolar disorder can be a great teacher. It's a challenge, but it can set you up to be able to do almost anything else in your life"

~Carrie Fisher

29:
Psychosis

The first three rounds of stem cells, with the addition of Prednisone, sent me into a full psychotic break. Prednisone can worsen bipolar disorder. This night was described at the beginning of this book with an account of the experience that landed me in the psych ward. Sadly, antibiotics can also cause mania in undiagnosed bipolar patients. The condition is called Antibiomania.

Even sadder, because it exceeded CDC guidelines, none of my antibiotic treatment was covered by my medical insurance. Neither was my stem cell or exosome treatments. Overall, we paid at least $100,000 out of pocket to save my life.

The night I walked down the street (and eventually ended up in the psych ward), I realized I was finally able to walk a full mile. Even though my mental health had plummeted from treatment, my physical strength seemed to be improving.

Antimicrobial-induced mania or antibiomania is rare and classified in the DSM-5 as "drug-induced manic episodes"

(Carrasco et al, 2002). Sadly, little is known as to what is the clinical demonstration, standard sufferer's characteristics, or mechanism of action for this syndrome. The consequences are real however, and with an increase in prescriptive medications being recommended, the probability of increased mania from antibiotics will increase correspondingly.

Cases reported include symptoms of increased "psychomotor activity, irritability, logorrhoea, hyperthymic mood, and difficulty falling asleep, as well as auditory hallucinations, mood-congruent mystical delusions, and delusions of harm (Carrasco et al, 2002). Testing on other systems, to include imaging and blood work, were normal and consistent with patients' ages, lack of comorbidity (including mental illness), and evidence of illicit or recreational substance use absent from findings. Upon cessation of the antibiotics, improvement to complete ending of symptoms were noted. These authors (2002) concluded a probable reaction to antibiotics taken by the patients.

Knowing the possibility of antibiomania resulting from long-term and frequent use of antibiotics allows victims of these types of episodes to look for other causes outside of mental health problems. It behooves those who suffer from these types of symptoms to advocate for answers that lie outside of additional medication administration, particularly another antibiotic.

In rehab, I continued with exosome treatment. Exosomes are part of a relatively new science that is a smaller component of stem cells—one that that can cross the blood-brain barrier. I did intra-nasal and IV exosomes and elected to skip the Prednisone during these treatments. I tolerated this well and did so without any negative psychological effects.

30:
Group Revelation

I also experienced the delusions and found myself handcuffed in the backseat of the police car.

"You don't understand," I said to a young girl walking past me with towels in her hands. "It's not my fault. It's the damn tick bite."

She didn't look at me.

No one looked at me. I was invisible once again—a number: 5250 and a resident in the psych ward.

"She's been here for over two weeks—sixteen days, to be exact. I think it's time for rehab," the psychologist announced.

"You're thinking Bipolar I disorder?"

"Yes, with psychosis," his associate said, nodding his head.

While in the hospital, it was announced that Covid had been designated a pandemic. Thankfully, the lesions on my skin began to clear up, likely from the stem cell treatment. Along with the healing skin, my hair began to grow back, all over my head without alopecia (missing) sections—also likely due to the stem cell treatments.

Again, no one talked to me about my situation, no one consulted with me about the decisions being made on my behalf.

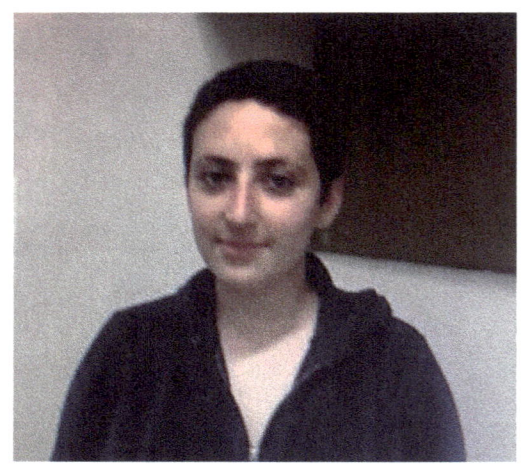

Intake photo for rehab in La Jolla 2020

The rehab lasted eight months. I started at a residential treatment level, even though I was still delusional and stabilizing from the Latuda. The physicians disagreed with the hospital's decision to put me on antipsychotics only, and decided I needed a mood stabilizer as well. This is when I was given Depakote.

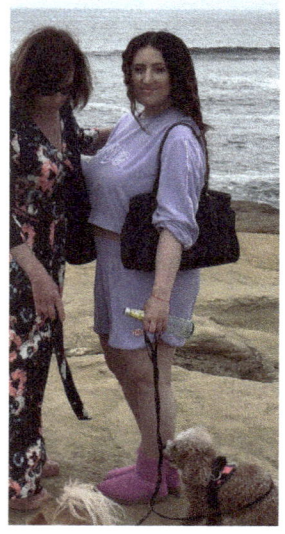

I already weighed 200 pounds and though Depakote can cause significant weight gain, the decision had been made for me. In the next few months, I gained another 35 pounds. Adding insult to injury, my insulin resistance was already triggered without any treatment or consideration. Of course, the psychiatric medications added to this issue.

30: Group Revelation

"I don't like how much weight I've gained recently. I don't feel good either," I said one day.

The nurse practitioner nodded and gave me a depreciating look, glancing at the obvious weight sitting in my body. "Maybe try a salad from Trader Joe's," she replied.

I was forced to sit in on AA meetings and read the Blue Book from Alcoholics Anonymous. Mainly, this was because there were no separate activities for people with mental health issues. The whole plan was by default but I had little choice at that point.

At first, I turned up my nose but decided to make the most of it and ended up really enjoying stories people shared about turning their lives around and doing the best they could on a day-by-day (sometimes minute-by-minute) basis. A few in rehab became good friends.

My program took me through two months of residential, next to PHP (a partial hospitalization program), and then to IOP (intensive outpatient program). My day consisted of daily group sessions, journaling, meditating, breath work, and therapy that I likely needed. It seemed I needed to rewire my brain after Lyme disease—even if the psychotic break and bipolar disorder hadn't happened. On the upside, this therapy plan gave me an outlet to process the loss of friendships, work through the medical PTSD, my body changes, and grieve the loss of the life I had anticipated for myself had I not gotten sick.

The first place I attended for residential treatment unexpectedly exposed a problem for me—I made the mistake in opening up about some of my delusions. One of the girls who, sadly, was an addict brought up my history, shared with her in confidence. Details of what I had told her were relayed in group therapy in front of one of the facilitators. I believe her goal was to embarrass me into realizing my thoughts were not reality. She had me backed into a corner because I was still deeply dealing with active delusions and felt the need to defend myself. Perhaps, she thought she was being helpful. But her action only embarrassed and shamed me.

Fortunately, not long after that event, I realized I was feeling much better physically. I experienced only one day of full body pain once, when we went to a park, and the advisors were compassionate enough to turn the car around and allow me to return to bed and recover. Still, I viewed this as a huge success and extreme improvement, after three years of lying in bed.

With prolonged and/or frequent use, Doxycycline is known for causing damage to teeth. I was no exception, as my teeth gradually turned black and green, and holes developed in the enamel. Multiple attempts to fix the problem, with the aid of a dentist, resulted in nothing but frustration. Something was not right. My teeth were grey and my gums were swollen and puffy.

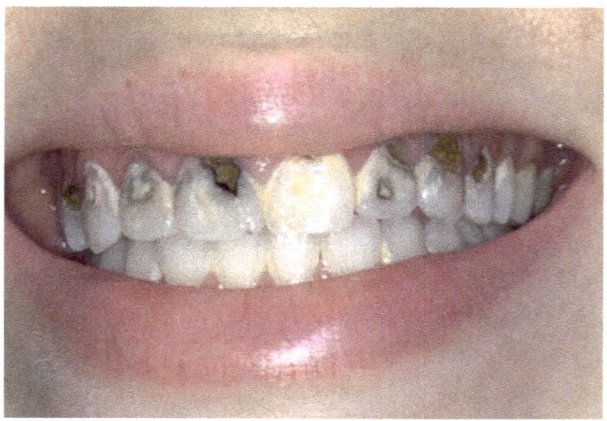

"You'll likely need crowns on the front six teeth, at the very least," the dentist said.

"That's not an option," I replied and sought other answers after leaving his office.

30: Group Revelation

Eventually, I would find a biological dentist who specialized in Lyme disease. She said we could fix most of my teeth through minimal-shaved veneers placed on my front six teeth and using a laser on my gums. "We can bleach the rest and give you back your amazing smile," she stated, her own brilliantly white teeth sparkling through a very caring smile. I trusted in her confidence and opted to move ahead with the treatment, which we did. My teeth have never looked better.

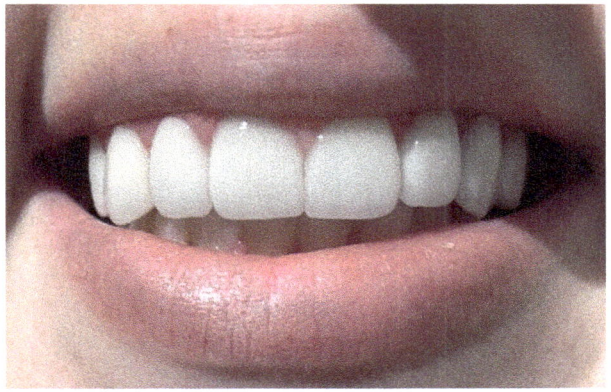

After all this time, it appeared that the stem cell and IV antibiotic therapy were healing my body, even though the treatment flared inflammation in my brain. But, I had a beautiful smile and that seemed to help a little.

31:
It's All on the Internet

The Latuda made me extremely groggy. But that wasn't as bad as the Depakote, which numbed my emotions until I barely recognized myself.

I allowed my parents to visit at this point (up until then, I had been extremely angry with them for the manner in which the 5150 occurred… and the trauma it caused). They frantically tried to tell me I was overly medicated.

"My parents noticed it when they visited me recently."

"I'm not sure you are ready for medicinal alterations, just yet, Kaitlyn." The doctor smiled as he spoke.

I swallowed back emotion and tried to sound reasonable and logical with an argument I would make up as I went. "I understand. My judgement is limited, but I should not be this sedated."

He smiled again, this time it looked genuine and less acerbic. "Mmm-hmmm."

"Look, I know this is a big request. But my parents know me. They've watched my progress, or lack of it… you could say… for most of my life. I trust their judgement and am asking that you do the same. Please. We can always go back to what you're giving me now, if they're wrong."

I had his attention.

He nodded and agreed with my plan. Within 24 hours, they started to wean me off of the Depakote. Slowly but surely, my joy returned, as did my personality. Sleep followed, and I found that I could fall asleep earlier than before when I was taking such a large dose of antipsychotics.

Staying alert wasn't exactly easy. Often, I would nearly drift off or my eyes would tear up for the second half of required evening classes because it was such a struggle to stay awake.

While in rehab, everyone was required to wear gloves and masks when running errands—this was during the COVID-19 pandemic. As most people struggled with isolation at that time, the same was not true for me. Every day in rehab, my association with people proved to be a blessing. This was the most socialization I had had in over three years.

Those days, I became close with one of the rehab workers—our connection to run errands together. She took me to shop for healthy food and encouraged me to cook. She was an addict who had been through a traumatic event, as well, and had also shaved her head. We had that in common. Fortunately, she was doing much better working a job and finding herself again.

I looked up to her.

One interesting characteristic about her—she was well versed on conspiracy theories. This allowed me to talk about some of my delusions and beliefs at the time without being shamed. I appreciated this friendship so much at that time.

I began to gradually realize that some of my delusions held no truth. It was like my mind was rewiring itself and bringing my thoughts back to reality. Sometimes, I cried and felt grief when I woke back up to the truth. I also felt extremely embarrassed at how I had publicly discussed some of them on my social media accounts that had many followers. Sadly, it was during that time that my influencer "reach" dwindled

31: It's All on the Internet

proportionate to my delusions. I did not keep up with the many changes taking place on many social media platforms, and began to fear being on social media, particularly after embarrassing myself there. I didn't hop on other social media trends, as a result, and let my exposure die down for a couple of years while I allowed myself to heal.

Truthfully, I enjoyed the quiet.

32:
Heiress Apparent

I planned to ship my new horse to California from Virginia but there were shipping regulations in place from the pandemic that prevented her from being shipped. So, we paid for her to stay in Virginia until the shipping laws would allow for her to come over. It eventually happened in July.

I received photo updates from her breeder and knew I needed to be my best self, physically and mentally. This became a necessary priority to be able to raise and train a baby horse. The responsibility was overwhelming to think about, but I felt motivated to get out and be better. She gave me something to look forward to.

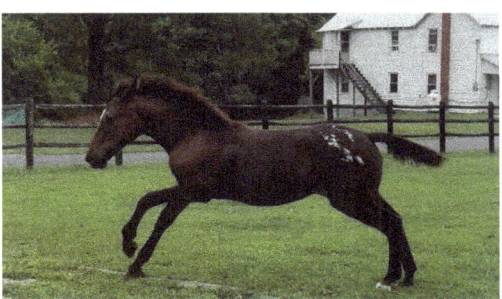

Photo Credit- Trinity Appaloosa Farm

Even though I had delusional episodes at that time of purchase, I still believe this horse was meant to be in my life and help me to heal. In July, while still in rehab, the COVID livestock shipping regulations lifted and I found a place for her 30 minutes from the rehab in Rancho Santa Fe. Every day, I would drive my car to visit this quiet, baby horse.

About this time, I started to struggle with Vasovagal Syncope/POTS without an official diagnosis. Yet, I would stand for long periods of time to visit her, even if that meant only 15 minutes at a time. Often, I would just check on her and then go back to bed and sleep.

Once, a POTS incident occurred when at Target. It called for emergent action and the tech with us almost called the ambulance. It was hot and I almost passed out standing in the long "social distancing" line waiting my turn to enter the store. I sat down and drank water and, after a while, recovered. This was the start of POTS worsening.

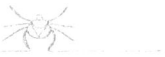

Postural orthostatic tachycardia syndrome or POTS is a syndrome characterized by rapid heartbeat (over 100 bpm) when moving from sitting or lying to standing position (orthostatic). The body's autonomic nervous system that typically manages blood pressure and heart rate doesn't kick in and cannot balance the changes that take place when the body's position changes. Symptoms such as dizziness, rapid pulse (tachycardia) or palpitations, nausea, fainting (syncope), exhaustion, shortness of breath (dyspnea), headaches, chest pain, and more can result. Not all of these symptoms are necessary to diagnose POTS. But a combination of medical history, along with any of the symptoms mentioned above, along with tests to determine what exactly is the cause will help establish a POTS diagnosis.

Causes are varied and are still being determined through research. However, many of those individuals who suffer from POTS share commonalities that can include women (ages <50 years), although men also suffer from POTS, stress, illnesses such as mononucleosis, pregnancy, trauma, surgery, autoimmune conditions (EBV, Sjogren's syndrome, lupus, etc.), even Lyme disease (Cleveland Clinic, 2022).

Each case of POTS is different. People with POTS may see symptoms come and go over a period of years. In most cases, with adjustments in diet, medications and physical activity, a person with POTS will experience an improvement in their quality of life (Cleveland Clinic, 2022).

Suffering from the symptoms associated with POTS is never pleasant. If you experience any of these symptoms, you should be assessed by your physician or present to an emergency department for further evaluation.

33:
Weight Peak and Back to School

"Congratulations!" they all said and handed me a certificate. I had finally graduated rehab. It was time to move back home.

At 235 pounds, it became evident that the next challenge to tackle was my weight. So, I reached out to a combined therapist and psychiatrist team. This therapist became my confidant and one of the best advocates I would have. She helped me tremendously to feel like myself again—one of my greatest blessings.

It was September 2020, and the feeling that I was still a shell of myself remained. Thankfully, my hair had been growing back, but that did nothing to help me recognize my body. It would be a process to "get there." So, I decided to take a risk and enroll back in school to finish my bachelor's degree—one class at a time. I added a second major in sociology and launched my education slowly, with the aid of a tutor.

"You're at 240 pounds now." This doctor didn't mince words and I knew I had to take my weight seriously.

"Oh," I replied. "I guess I'll go back on a diet."

There was no response from the doctor who kept his eyes glued to the notes he was making in my chart. The next day, I started a diet program again. It had worked for me when in high school, maybe it would work again.

The food was much worse than I remembered. The portions were tiny and I felt like I was starving myself. After a while, I quit. So, the hunt for another weight-reduction program ensued. Another company caught my eye. The food was keto-based with shakes three times daily, bars, and veggies and protein added in whenever possible. A Styku body scan was performed and my result horrified me. I was considered a very high percentage for risk. The health issues and the body image didn't align with how I wanted to look. None of it came close to how I saw myself in my mind.

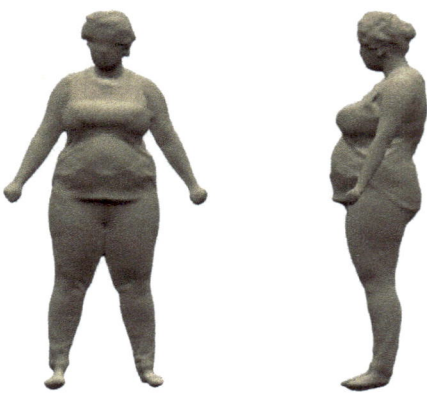

Styku body scan at highest weight

In the first week, I dropped eight pounds. Hope was the result. Then the plateau hit and my weight loss stalled. Rather than the health coach suggesting a medical issue, she immediately took a different stance.

33: Weight Peak and Back to School

"I think… well, let's just say that it's obvious you must not be following the program." Her hands rested on her hips and I felt like a five-year-old in trouble for cutting the lunch line.

"I don't cheat! I follow the plan religiously." My response sounded childish, but I spoke the truth.

"Anything you put into your mouth that isn't in your plan will cause added weight—even a couple of pounds," she replied.

That hit home. I had, indeed, put on another two pounds that week.

Not long after that, the store closed for good. I had lost a total of 15 pounds with the program but faced another turn of bad luck.

34:
Mediterranean Diet

Restrictive is an understatement!

The most recent program offered food that wasn't palpable and scant in calories, both of which were bad for my mental health. It taught about good and bad foods and made it clear that if one cheated in any way, they would lose all progress made for that week. It felt like a penal code passed down through food.

It was time to act and find another way to deal with my weight issues. So, I found an endocrinologist and called a bariatric surgeon. I was sick of living like this in this body—one that I hardly recognized. They tested my insulin level, which came back too high and that led to an official diagnosis of "insulin resistance" with a new medication: metformin. None of this helped to lose the weight. Still, it didn't increase and could be classified as "stable."

Next, I met a nutritionist that helped me to establish a healthy relationship with food again. She believed the Mediterranean was the best diet around. She encouraged fruits and vegetables and allowed whole grains again—something the previous program had banned. A personal trainer was also suggested, one that would understand my medical conditions. I found the perfect trainer in Bob Kelly, Jr.

The nutritionist allowed a small "cheat" cup of ice cream once a week. This approach proved successful for me mentally, and I followed the 1200 calorie meal plan for months. However, only five pounds came off.

"Gosh, this works for other people," she apologized. "I can't understand why you're not losing weight."

I had no response and merely shrugged. I liked her and the plan she had for me. And while all of the weight didn't come off, the lifestyle set me up to be successful in the future.

The benefit of the Mediterranean Diet is not new. In fact, physicians have touted its benefit for cardiovascular health for years. Whole, organic, and healthy omega-rich foods are the basis of the diet, a standard way of eating in Mediterranean regions. These foods include, according to U. C. Davis Health (2024):

- Fruits and vegetables
- Nuts and seeds, including almonds, walnuts, sunflower seeds, and pumpkin seeds
- Beans and legumes, such as lentils, chickpeas, black beans, and kidney beans
- Whole grains like whole wheat bread, quinoa, brown rice, and whole wheat pasta
- Fish and seafood
- Healthy fats and oils, including extra virgin olive oil and avocado and nut oils

The benefits include not just cardiovascular health, but also, decreased risk for cancer, improved cognition and mental health, improvement to diabetes and other illnesses, as well as symptoms of Lyme disease.

34: Mediterranean Diet

Functional health wellness advocates often use micronutrient testing to identify how diet can be used to improve those suffering from symptoms related to Lyme:

> The SpectraCell Micronutrient Test is a comprehensive blood test that measures the levels of various vitamins, minerals, antioxidants, and other essential nutrients within an individual's cells. This test can help identify specific nutrient deficiencies that may be contributing to ongoing inflammation, fatigue, and cognitive issues often associated with this condition (Yoshimura, H., 2025).

Whole, organic foods rich in antioxidants and vitamins Bs, C, and D are particularly beneficial for a weakened immune system, as is the case for those suffering from Lyme.

The admonition that "Food is medicine" (Melville, 2024), is well-remembered when considering what can be done as a first step to mitigate the debilitating symptoms of chronic Lyme disease.

35:
With the Help of GLP-1 Medications

"You really don't qualify for bariatric surgery on your own," the surgeon announced. "You need at least two comorbidities for me to operate. Unfortunately, simply being a hundred pounds overweight won't cut it."

His comments blew my mind! Our meeting went against the nutritionist's advice, but I had to find out for myself what the options were. I looked into the lap band procedure, which currently is being phased out.

"What else can I do, then?" I asked in response.

"Well, the healthiest, and the safest, procedure is the gastric sleeve. If your cholesterol is high and we can identify one other issue, you can get approved for weight loss surgery."

"My cholesterol is high," I confessed.

"Maybe the next step is to meet with a medical weight loss doctor."

He was finished with me… but I hadn't given up just yet.

I called my endocrinologist and asked if she knew of any medications that could help me lose weight—any medications that were *not* stimulants.

"I'm afraid not. I won't write you any weight loss prescriptions due to your bipolar diagnosis."

"I see."

"Truthfully, I'm not impressed with your progress on metformin."

I swallowed and tried to keep my composure. "Me neither," I said and she added, "I think you need bariatric surgery. I honestly don't believe you will lose the weight without it."

She studied me for a moment then I said I'd think about it.

At our next appointment, she stated wanted bariatric surgery scheduled.

"My understanding is that I'm not heavy enough," I said, explaining the information given to me by the bariatric surgeon.

"Well, then you'll just have to gain more weight!" my endocrinologist announced.

My face blanched and I had no words. Apparently, she noticed because she immediately added, "Or you can just embellish some comorbidity to get qualified. You know what I mean."

I swallowed back the shock and mentioned that I had done some research on the subject. "The surgeon told me I had options, something outside of stimulants. I'll just follow up with a medical weight loss doctor first and see what they think about it."

She nodded. I guess she had no other suggestions.

The weight loss doctor proved beneficial and prescribed me Wegovy for treatment. I took my first injection November 8, 2021. Thankfully, the GLP-1 medications would help get my physical body back on track.

The first few months of this medication was wonderful. I wondered if this was what a *normal person's* brain felt like. I had always been obsessive about food and wondered when and what my next meal would be. I learned that this obsession is called "food noise." With the Wegovy, the noise was gone. I

35: With the Help of GLP-1 Medications

was able to eat what I wanted in moderation—still choosing healthy, for the most part, by staying on a 1200 calorie diet. My body responded to the medication.

I lost weight.

I began to feel so much better about myself mentally and physically. I was doing well on Wegovy and felt some relief about the whole situation. However, that didn't last long. Once the dose was increased to 1.7 mg., I began to vomit multiple times a day. The doctor dropped my dose back to 1 mg with hopes that it would mitigate the nausea and vomiting, but after only a week, I still vomited.

"I don't think Wegovy is the right drug for you," the doctor announced.

I stopped Wegovy March 21, 2022. This was very upsetting because I could see it worked and my weight was down to 180 pounds. Within a month after stopping the Wegovy, my weight increased five pounds and along with it, the hunger and food noise.

"Let's try Topamax," the doctor suggested next.

But my urine turned hazy and was painful. In addition, there was a sensation of numbness and tingling in my hands and feet. This created an unsafe situation for me to drive like this. I felt uncomfortable with it, and I put on another two pounds.

The situation worsened. I had to find answers but once again, they eluded me.

I went on the Tick Boot Camp podcast and told my story (episode 199). During a 90 minute interview, my history was shared and my experience with Lyme became public. I was a little hesitant because I still didn't yet feel or look like myself, but podcaster Freddie Kimmel told me, "You never know if your story is going to be the magic that someone needs to hear in order to heal." That resonated with me.

So, I decided to participate.

I made more 'Lyme friends' throughout this process and joined Lyme disease support groups. My hope was that one day I would be able to elaborate even further on my story.

36:
Back to One-der-land

"Well, at 5' 5" in height, 180 pounds really isn't that fat. I wouldn't worry about it and just find a way to live with it."

"But that's not…"

"You'll never see 135 pounds again," the weight loss doctor stated. "And besides, it's not really a healthy goal for you."

"Why?"

"Honestly, I think your best weight goal should be 155 pounds. It's really the lowest weight you're likely to see, anyway, at this point," the weight loss doctor said.

"I'm not happy with those numbers."

"Well, if you're not happy at 180 pounds, you'll never be happy here. Maybe you should move to another state, like Arkansas. You'll be skinny there."

This was not an option for me, neither was her suggestion to move. It was unacceptable and inappropriate, and I fell back to being my own best resource.

The word about semaglutide medications spread as a hot "weight loss" option. The result was a Wegovy shortage. I begged the weight loss doctor to allow a lower dose just to stay on the medicine, even to increase dosages at a slower rate. This was something I'd learned worked for people in a Facebook support group I had joined.

"Well, I'll agree to a 0.25 mg. dose for weight maintenance but no more."

"Deal!" was my enthusiastic reply.

Sadly, Wegovy was nowhere to be found. I felt defeated and a bit manipulated by the suggestion. So again, I opted for a new course of action. I called my primary doctor next.

"I'm interested in trying Ozempic. I understand it has the same active ingredients as Wegovy, and since that's unavailable, I thought that Ozempic might be a good option." My primary care doctor gave no response, so I continued. "Look, I've had positive results from semaglutide medications and just want to stay consistent with something that I know works."

His response was positive and I followed up with the next available appointment they offered. He agreed to let me stay on a low dose and increase slowly by counting clicks, if needed. This med was approved by the insurance company, as well. Everything fell into place—a positive way forward.

I started Ozempic on May 5, 2022. Following the doctor's suggestion to start with a low dose and gradually increase as needed, I didn't face any side effects from the Wegovy, including vomiting. The combination of medication, diet, and exercise with my trainer led to weight loss. By July 17, 2023, I had dropped to 134 pounds—one pound under my goal weight—a total of over *one hundred pounds* lost without any surgery.

This was an incredible accomplishment—to beat the odds and do what the doctors had told me was impossible. My endocrinologist apologized and admitted that I'd proved her wrong and needed to write a book talking about my experience—so I did!

36: Back to One-der-land

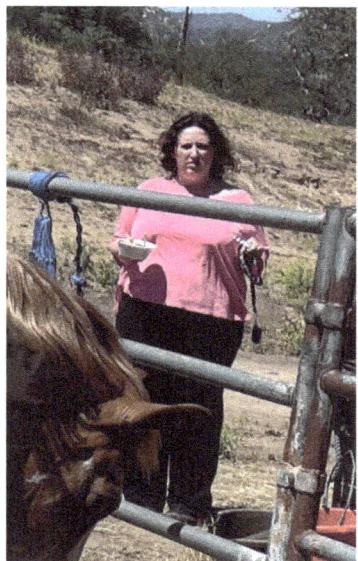 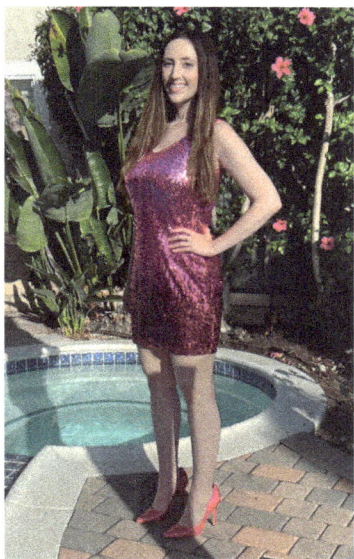

Pre- and Post-Weight Loss of 105 lbs.

With the help of GLP-1 medications I was able to reverse the inflammation from Lyme disease, as well as the steroid weight gain. It was true, what my LLMD had said: "You never had an obesity problem, you had an inflammation problem. The medications reverse inflammation." He suggested I stay on them long-term. I couldn't agree more!

With personal training, healthy eating habits, and GLP-1 medication (to include metformin), I had reached my pre-Lyme and steroid goal weight. Most importantly, I felt great.

37:
Bachelor's Degree at Last

A new LLMD was recommended by a family friend the following January. He took my entire history and re-diagnosed me with MCAS, POTS, and (after palpating my neck) said that I had a concussion and possibly traumatic brain injury (TBI). This could have occurred when, in second grade, I hit my head in the pool. Or it might have happened the time I hit my head on a slip-n-slide at band camp.

"Well, Epstein Barr is probably the least of your worries, but we can address it," the doctor said and arranged for me to have IV therapy two to three times a week. IV NAD+, glutathione, B12, and hydration were prescribed.

A few months into treatment, he became suspicious that I still had lingering Lyme. I paid for a new Lyme (with coinfections) test that took six weeks for the primary results to come back. This test showed multiple positive bands of a European strain of Lyme, and so, the physician gave me another Lyme diagnosis. My bartonella test was elevated but not clinically positive. Still, he was suspicious of lingering bartonella as well. All other tick-borne infections were negative. He ran a full virus panel and I tested positive for many.

"Well, your lab results are lit up like a Christmas tree," the doctor announced.

I wasn't surprised.

I graduated with a 3.8 GPA in my last two years of college and was able to walk in two ceremonies for my college graduation. The same academic advisor whose mother had Lyme disease had returned after retiring just to run the smaller ceremony for the psychology department. I walked up to her and reminded her of who I was and briefly rehearsed my story, after which she gave me a "high-five" and then embraced me, bear-hug style—proud that I had accomplished so much against the odds. I was equally proud, along with her, that I had stuck it out and returned to finish my education. My freshman year social psychology professor was also there, receiving his own award, and I had the opportunity to say "hello" to him, as well. This felt like a special, full-circle, meant-to-be moment for me.

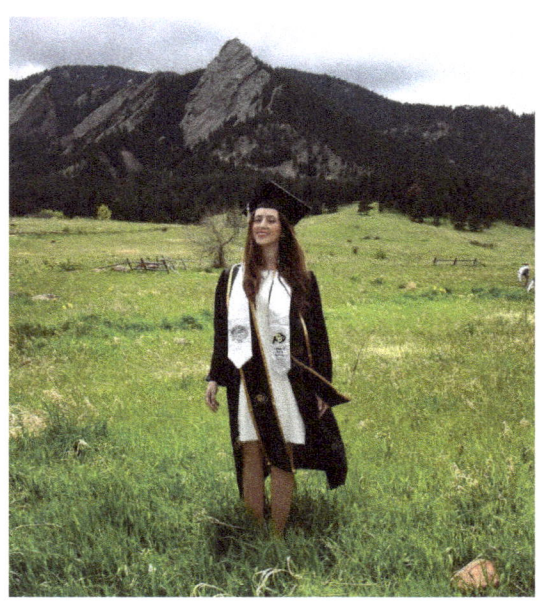

38:
Grad School

My application was accepted for entry into a master's degree program. I decided at that time to pursue a graduate degree in forensic psychology (court psychology) to learn the legal system with the hopes of supporting victims of Lyme disease who also suffer from mental health issues through my influence. My intent is to make crisis intervention less traumatic for those who experience mental illness and spread awareness about Lyme and mental health. So much about mental health care needs to be improved, such as including a social worker in all mental health calls to ensure the safety of both the person in crisis and also the first responders.

I believe that if a program had been implemented to include a social worker, and had been part of my city's program, my experience would have been less traumatic. According to one new published study, patients with psychotic disorder are "three times more likely to have Bartonella DNA in their blood than adults without these disorders. The work further supports the idea that pathogens—particularly vector-borne pathogens—could play a role in mental illness." (Peake, 2024).

A relatively new term coined the psychiatric effects and results of Lyme's effect on mental health: "neuropsychiatric

Lyme." This is currently being discussed in journal articles. Mental illness has a biological component that's been previously missed. Now, is the time, more importantly than ever, to study Lyme disease and its effects on mental health. A Harvard study states the following:

> These infections are behind the blood brain barrier and inside human neurons. Borrelia biofilms are commonly and routinely seen as embedded aggregates inside amyloid plaques that are seen in Alzheimer's brains that we have studied. We studied 112 brains from the bank at Harvard University, of 5/5 autopsied Alzheimer infected brains also showed Lyme Spirochetes further proving the effect of Lyme on mental health and brain health (Grier, 2019).

After graduation, I returned home to learn of the final results of the lab tests. The physician and I discussed whether or not I wanted another port or Hickman catheter and to try IV antibiotics. I didn't. My request was for another option.

"Since you're stable, I think you are a good candidate for LDN," the physician said. This is low-dose naltrexone, which when used in microdoses treats Lyme. He suggested we do this in combination with herbal tincture treatment. He added, "The herbs can be brutal but we will go slowly."

Nothing could be as bad as my experience with IV antibiotics, so I was willing to naltrexone a try.

To my surprise, the herbs proved to be a better outcome for me. Many are herbal tinctures from *Beyond Balance*, an herbal store that I trust. Their products can be found through their website: https://beyondbalanceinc.com.

38: Grad School

Currently, we are treating Lyme, Bartonella, and all of the viruses that lit-up on my blood work. The brain inflammation is being managed with "cognease detox." We also do microcurrent therapy to stimulate my vagus nerve and improve my POTS. My heart rate is finally in a normal range for the first time since college. I will treat with herbs fully for at least nine months and then reevaluate. Mold exposure is being treated with Vitamin C and binders.

With these new treatments, I am improving. My activity level is tremendously improved: going to concerts, theme parks, on boat rides, traveling, riding my horse multiple times weekly, etc. I am succeeding in grad school and making new friends. I haven't found my "person" yet, but hopefully that is in my future. I would like children one day, as well. I know that for this to happen, I need my Lyme levels to be as low as possible… hopefully nonexistent and in complete remission.

A girl can dream.

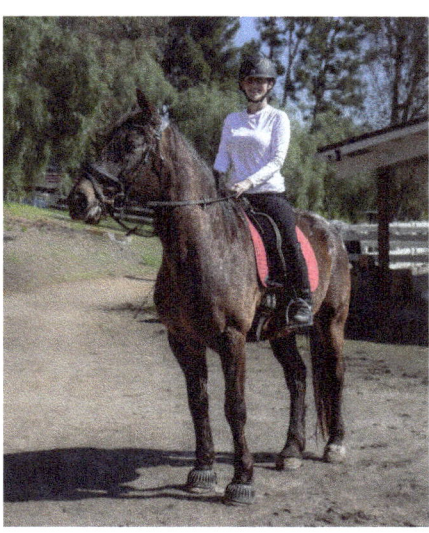

Chantilly age 6

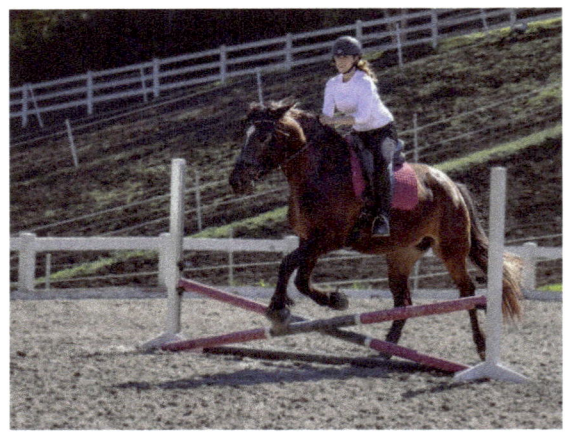

I am not at 100% remission yet but my current wellness situation gives me hope, knowing that I have room to improve. Under the current treatment, I feel 90% healed. Soon, a recheck of my C6 peptide will see if Lyme is still active, in the slightest. My mental health has been stable for almost five years... so much so that my therapist, psychiatric nurse, and Lyme doctor all doubt an organic bipolar diagnosis—instead believing it was a secondary bipolar due to Lyme disease. In the meantime, I stay on a low dose Latuda (a psych medication), for now.

My Lyme doctor jokes that the average person on the street takes at least two psych meds, so I am doing great! I do not have ups, downs, or any symptoms of bipolar any longer. Those events are a distant memory. With therapy, I have learned to regulate my emotions and can communicate calmly and effectively. Back then, I could barely string a full sentence together. That was at my worst, but now I am thriving in Grad school with the hopes of graduating "with distinction" (my school's term for a 4.0 grade point average). I was invited to join my school's of Psi Chi, The International Honor Society in Psychology.

38: Grad School

In addition, my weight is stable at around 135 pounds. This has been so for a couple years. I have come off of Metformin and am just maintaining with a lower, maintenance dose of Ozempic. My hope is that my story also gives you, the reader, a sense of hope and the promise that Lyme disease does not have to define you.

This is a disease that may have started with a little bug but is managed by the power of the human will—a will to live a healthy, full life.

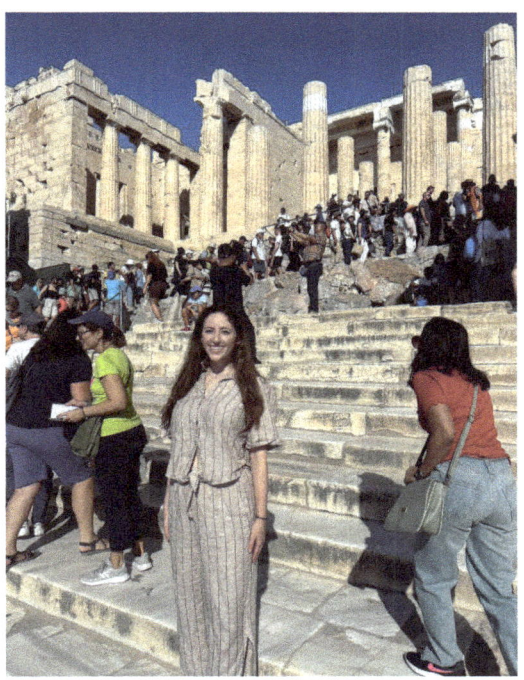

Traveling the world- Athens, Greece 2023

39:
The Board of Pharmacy

Someone informed me that the California Board of Pharmacy was working to ban Category I compounds including my treatments Glutathione, NAD+, and methyl cobalamin—the activated form of vitamin B12. I knew I needed to help. A meeting was scheduled that requested public comments about the topic. I decided to share my story and bring light to the fact that many of these compounds are crucial for "Lyme Warriors." I spoke of how the compounded medications helped me during my Lyme disease journey and pleaded with the board to reconsider their planned and dangerous restrictions.

Not long afterward, the president of Lymedisease.org, Dorothy Kupcha Leland, contacted me. She was ready to fight to provide access to these medications for victims of Lyme.

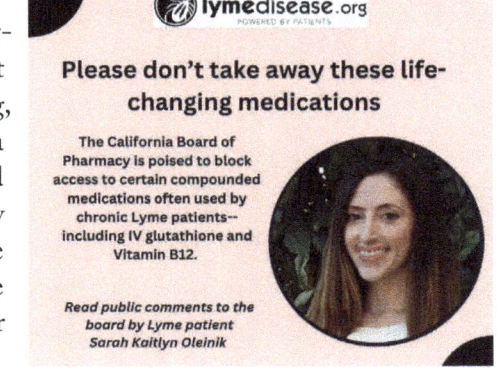

"We'd like a copy of your transcript from your presentation," she asked.

"Of course," I responded, and sent it over immediately. Not long afterward, I was contacted by her again, this time asking permission to do a write-up about me, and please provide a head shot. Again, I agreed and sent the requested photo.

My article was published August of 2024. I had stepped into the role of becoming an advocate.

For Your Information

"A man's accomplishments in life are the cumulative effect of his attention to detail."

~ John Foster Dulles, American Diplomat

FYI—Let's Talk About Options

"To heal Lyme disease, take some medicine, try some treatments, heal some trauma."

(Instagram @thetickchicks).

Finding an LLMD

If bitten or suspecting Lyme disease and based on the symptom tracking list, I highly recommend finding a Lyme-literate medical doctor to help you figure out what's going on with your body. This will be a journey. You can visit the ILAD's provider search: https://www.ilads.org/patient-care/provider-search/ for resources.

Remember, while in medical school, most medical doctors are only taught a very small segment about Lyme disease. As a result, physicians generally cannot recognize symptoms of Lyme disease and aren't sure what to do, especially should your presentation *not* include a history of a tick bite or the presentation of the obvious bull's-eye rash. Most doctors will prescribe a quick round of doxycycline but have little knowledge about co-infections such as:

- Bartonella/Bartonellosis
- Ehrlichia/Ehrlichiosis

- Anaplasma/Anaplasmosis
- Rocky Mountain spotted fever (RMSF)
- Borrelia Miyamotoi
- Borrelia Mayonii
- Colorado Tick Fever
- Heartland Virus
- Powassan Virus
- Q Fever
- Relapsing Fever
- Southern Tick-Associated Rash Illness
- Tick-Borne Encephalitis
- Tularemia
- Brucellosis

Other side effects include:

- Tick Paralysis
- Alpha-Gal Meat Allergy

Source: Introducing Co-Infections - Project Lyme

Lyme is often not just Lyme. Especially when it hits the chronic phase, the disease can be triggered by an immune system response. This is believed to be why some people become chronically ill while others do not. Additional illnesses develop or are triggered, as a result, such as: PANS/PANDAS, MCAS, arthritis, and perhaps a previously existing Ehlers Danlos Syndrome. Having an integrative Lyme-literate physician (LLMD) that can look at the "big health picture" in relation to your symptoms is crucial to solving the Lyme disease puzzle. The downside is, LLMD practices usually do not accept insurance and generally have pricey consultation fees. It can also take some time to find a doctor with whom you agree and in whom you feel confident. Trial and error are crucial.

39: The Board of Pharmacy

If, for any reason, a doctor or the recommended treatment doesn't feel right, keep looking and try something else. Hopefully, as we continue to make our voices heard about Lyme as we educate the general population, and we make strides in legalizing Lyme, things will change. My current Lyme doctor is one of the few that does accept insurance. Even my weekly IV treatments are partially covered, which is extremely exciting and shows forward progress with the healthcare system.

Another option is to find a health coach to guide you through the process. Remember though, a coach is not legally able to give medical advice. Your coach can guide you to healing options or refer you to an herbalist or a natural medicine practitioner who takes a more natural route.

My first LLMD treated me too aggressively. My body couldn't handle her treatment at that time, but I am not sure I would be here, moving forward in the direction my body is going now if it weren't for meeting her. My current LLMD is listening to me, considering my past history, and taking a more natural approach using herbs.

Occasionally, doctors sell herbal kits or publicly list protocol recommendations, such as the Buhner Protocol from Stephen Burner's book, *Healing Lyme*, or Dr. Bill Rawl's, *Herbal Protocol*. These are good resources, in my opinion, if a doctor visit is completely out of the budget.

If you and your doctor decide that antibiotics are not the treatment for you, or you have tried them with no improvement, do not give up—there are plenty of other healing modalities to try: herbs, rife machine, IV therapy (such as glutathione, NAD+, B vitamins, vitamin C), energy healing, acupuncture, bee venom therapy, tens unit, parasite zapper, ozone treatments, stem cells, exosomes, stevia, colloidal silver, methylene blue, rife machine, opening up the drainage pathways, and Epsom salt baths, to name a few.

A list of alternative therapies can be found on the website: Alternative Treatment list from Lymedisease.org

Herbal protocols, sauna, chelation or detoxification treatments, medical marijuana, acupuncture, homeopath, nutraceuticals, electromagnetic energy therapy, hyperthermia or heat therapy, oxygen therapy (ozone, etc.), rife machine, colloidal silver, hyperbaric oxygen treatment, stem cell therapies, exosomes, and Psilocybin are often listed on the following sites:

Source: https://www.lymedisease.org/mylymedata-alternative-lyme-disease-treatment/

Psilocybin: https://pmc.ncbi.nlm.nih.gov/articles/PMC9990519/

In addition, new antibiotic combo therapies are being tested and researched every day, although these studies tend to *not* include chronically ill patients with ground-breaking treatments.

Mold Illness and Microbes: Mental Health

Delusions often happen before psychosis throws them completely out of control. It happened that way with me, and I often wish my family, friends, or LLMD had recognized the signs during the early stages. My belief is that a simple recognition of the symptoms would have saved me from the traumatic trip to the hospital (in a police car), followed by a distressing sixteen-day stay in a psych ward.

It's not the medical professional's fault—this information isn't taught in med school, health classes, or even discussed openly. Sadly, self-awareness goes out the window when someone is in the depths of a psychotic event. The delusions feel real. One's psychotic experience prevents rational thought and the individual cannot determine what is *in their head* versus what is reality.

39: The Board of Pharmacy

I suffered with both auditory and an inner monologue constantly running delusional thoughts during psychosis. I had moments, such as considering the need for a brain scan, to get clarity and the reassurance that something was seriously wrong with me.

None of it was enough to turn off the racing, delusional thoughts.

I hope that by discussing what led up to my psychosis and by illuminating what others experience, before a large psychotic break, will help prevent the same from happening to others. If someone you know with Lyme is experiencing mental health issues, I strongly recommend a Lyme therapist and psychiatrist as professional team members, in addition to an LLMD. There are more and more Lyme-literate therapists and psychiatrists coming out in the field who are willing to discuss mental illness, Lyme, mold illness, and coinfections.

A new study has found that patients diagnosed with schizophrenia, or another psychotic disorder, are three times more likely to have *Bartonella* DNA in their blood than adults without these disorders (Peak, T. (2024).

The findings are significant and can mean the difference between misdiagnosis and proper treatment.

When losing myself to delusion, the roof above my bedroom leaked and likely filled with mold. We later tested the house and found that black mold had been growing in our downstairs bathroom, as well as other kinds of mold in different places in the house.

I recommend testing for mold if psychiatric illness is playing a role in those types of symptoms. Other indicators are confusion, racing thoughts, mood swings, decreased hygiene, change in sleep patterns, intense emotions or a lack thereof. I often sent manic lengthy emails to my physician that she noted were disorganized and paranoid. She didn't have time to read them to know what they meant. I wish she had recognized that this new behavior indicated illness. I also had little emotional capacity or tolerance for ER doctors and would speak harshly to them whenever I needed to go to the hospital. My mental capacity affected how I was treated at these times, which isn't right but is an unfortunate consequence of the current medical system.

Once, I was dismissed as hysterical when actually, I was dealing with sepsis. After reviewing my blood tests hours later, the hospital called back in a panic with a frantic, new plan of care.

Mold illness can be diagnosed through urine tests and advanced blood tests. LLMD's are aware of these tests and have access to arranging this specialized testing for their patients. At-home mold tests can be ordered, as well, and sent to a lab to determine the specific mold species and bacteria that are growing in your home. My current LLMD recommends "Immunolytics Plates" to place around the home.

Before slipping into full-blown psychosis, I grew more and more isolated, snapping at friends and losing relationships on all sides. I couldn't physically see anyone other than my home health care nurses and parents due to immunodeficiency, brain swelling, being sensitive to sound, and unable to walk most days. This went on for a couple of years, adding to the increasing isolation. My friends stopped calling to check on me. I had no visitors. Fortunately, the few friends with Lyme disease that connected through social media became the people I relied on most during this time.

I felt extremely alone and embarrassed with my mental health, but the more Lyme warriors I connected with, the more I realized my story was not unique. This is still true to this day, and the reason I share my story—to break the stigma. I have met many other Lyme warriors dealing with

Lyme-triggered bipolar, 5150's, police calls, Baker Acts, PANS/PANDAS, and more.

The evolving term for this psychosis is *Neuropsychiatric Lyme*.

Suicide is a huge issue in the Lyme community, as well. People are frequently told they are "going crazy" by doctors, as their symptoms are dismissed. And then, from a psychiatric standpoint, the patient has the feeling they really are losing their mind.

Mental health support is crucial to dealing with Lyme that has invaded one's brain.

Holistic psychologist, Judy S Tsafrir in an article written for *Psychology Today* (2017) recognizes the effects of mold toxicity on the body and its contribution to mental illness.

Toxic mold-based illness is a very prevalent and under diagnosed condition that can manifest in many different ways, including with symptoms that are exclusively psychiatric, such as depression, anxiety, attentional problems, brain fog and insomnia.

Common illness that is identified as generalized; classic mental illness is often a symptom of mold exposure. This needs to be explored in greater detail to prevent the same traumatic scenario as I experienced.

Had I an astute mental health team in place before treatment started, I could have prevented a lot of trauma… and a lot more heartache.

The Nose Knows

My nose runs incessantly! This has gone on for years and, honestly, I've been very frustrated living with it. It worsens when I put on my makeup or have something social to attend, like a date. Try as I might, there's never anything to blow out… then, all of a sudden, my nose pours like a faucet.

When I expressed my frustration to the doctor, he did not seem very concerned and replied, "Your runny nose is not my top priority." After complaining about it for a year, the doctor finally gave in. "I've heard you complain about this enough. We're going to swab your nose and send it out to a special lab. Let's see if they can identify what's causing this incessant rhinorrhea."

The results came back and revealed that I have Staphylococcus coag-negative (large amount) and MaRCoNs up in my nasal passages. I also have a small amount of monila sitophila, as well, which is a type of mold. This is common in people with *immunodeficiency, those on immunosuppressive drugs, and those with debilitating disease*, such as Lyme.

These symptoms are not exclusive to me. Should you suffer from the same symptoms, there is a test that your physician will order to determine what is the cause. The lab we used was Microbiology DX, INC. They run three types of tests off of one swab for $350. The fungal cultures will take one month to get the results.

More information can be found here: https://mylymedoc.com/is-marcons-contagious/

> Someone told me, **"If you don't make time for your wellness, your body will make time for your illness."**

Many believe that trauma stored in your body will trigger dis-ease, or disease, in the expressed as physical illness in the body. Many Lyme patients are type-A, high over-achievers. I overworked myself in school, striving for straight A's, spending consecutive days in the gym, socializing, and having zero tools to regulate my panic attacks before I relapsed from Lyme. I had taken an AP psychology class in high school and was a psychology major in college and still had no idea that the

39: The Board of Pharmacy

choices I made for myself could lead me to relapse from Lyme. I never realized that Lyme could be the root of my mental health issues. In truth, I did not know that relapsing was even possible because my primary care doctor had treated me, and I thought I had finished with that of my life.

Being able to take care of your body, regulate your emotions, and control the fight-or-flight response in the body can prevent autoimmune diseases and other illnesses (like Lyme) from relapsing. I currently stay in therapy every other week, not only to manage my bipolar diagnosis, but also to address my trauma. EMDR has allowed me to process and move past the traumatic events in life.

As they say, "Happy mind, happy body."

Healing my mind and learning the tools to have healthy appropriate reactions and responses to triggers has helped regulate my nervous system enough to heal my body. This is possible for anyone willing to put in the effort to heal.

Be wary, however, of substances and how they affect your mental health during treatment. The ADHD medication I had been taking for over ten years suddenly began to induce manic behavior. Marijuana is sometimes recommended for Lyme patients' treatment of pain, but that can worsen mental health issues and trigger psychosis and mania. Psychoactive treatments such as Ketamine or Psilocybin are not recommended for those who have experienced psychosis because there is a risk for getting trapped in that state.

If you suffer with mood changes, become paranoid, or begin to experience hallucinations, discuss it with your doctors immediately. I recommend you ask someone trustworthy to monitor your mood and check in with you frequently, as well as be willing to discuss how they think you are coping and dealing with Lyme treatment. This person will need to be honest when/if they see any changes in your personality.

Many of my friends distanced themselves rather than expressing their concern to my family. My doctor noticed changes but never suggested that I needed to see a psychiatrist, nor did she mention that she suspected the Lyme was worsening my mental health issues. In fact, she denied it. If she had acknowledged this, it could've saved me a lot of anguish.

Friendships

I lost many friendships during my illness. Author Kris Newby discusses an anomaly that involves someone who is diagnosed with cancer receiving casseroles from their neighbors. This is not typically the case for Lyme patients. Most people know nothing about Lyme, and because the disease typically presents as an "invisible illness," many times its victims are not believed.

The mental health symptoms triggered, such as Lyme rage, can cause people to overreact and to not behave like themselves. There is also something called the Herxheimer Reaction. I was not the exception to the above and rarely acted like myself when healing from Lyme disease. Often, I would snap at the people I loved the most. Between the inability to regulate my emotions and the onset of Lyme-triggered bipolar symptoms, I unintentionally pushed away those I loved, including the best friend I always considered a sister.

The advice I'd offer to friends of Lyme patients: Do not take the Lyme patient's behavior and actions personally. Know it is the illness and not your friend reacting out of character. Continue to invite your warrior friend out to events, even if the patient cannot attend. Doing so makes the Lyme warrior feel included and still a part of your life. Ask how the Lyme patient is really doing. When you are in the place and can hold space for the Lyme warrior to vent, let them know. It can be hard to hear about friends who have "wins" when the patient's

39: The Board of Pharmacy

life is on hold but know that the patient-warrior still wants to hear about your successes and cheer for you.

Christa Nannos, in her book, *Tick Tok It's Lyme O'Clock* dives deep into relationships and friendships and discusses how to navigate those relationships with Lyme. I highly recommend her book.

At first, I attempted to repair my original friendships after I made huge steps to progress in my healing, but I wasn't very successful in repairing these friendships. I hope this is not the case for you. I focused on moving forward and meeting new people—first turning to Lyme support groups to make friends with others who would understand my story. Due to limited energy, we first engaged in zoom movie nights to spend time together. Now that I am more active, I spend a lot of time at the barn with women my age and am beginning to get a normal social life back. It takes time, and that is okay. It is okay to mourn the life you once had. You will likely never get that back, but you can move forward and build a life that is more intentional and healthier moving forward.

Those meant to be in your life will stay. To the ones that leave, wish them well and allow them to exit. Mel Robbins discusses the "Let Them" theory. Let people show you who they are and how much they value you. If your friends go out to brunch without you… let them.

You get to choose on whom you focus in your life and into whom you pour your energy moving forward. Socializing with Lyme can be complicated and at times difficult, but you can figure out what works for you.

I do not drink as much as my peers, but often will sip on one drink throughout the night just to feel social. Some Lyme warriors cannot tolerate this. I recommend bringing our own drinks or food you tolerate and letting the host know it's not personal, just necessary for your health. You may also experience post-exertional malaise (as I did) where you might be in bed for one or two days after a social event. Only now, five years after stem cell therapy and IV antibiotics, is this getting better for me. This is also due to my current herbal treatment and low-dose naltrexone that helps to rid those last remaining levels of Lyme.

Make lemonade

Crisis events and situations can often be critical turning points in a person's life. They can serve as a challenge and opportunity for rapid problem resolution and growth, or as a debilitating event leading to sudden disequilibrium, failed coping, and dysfunctional behavior patterns (Roberts, 2005, p. xx).

The choice is yours! You have all the power.

You can let something that seems difficult make you or break you. I was first humiliated by my psychotic episode and didn't plan to tell a soul outside of my immediate family and the few friends I still trusted. However, when Matt and Rich asked me to be on the Tick Boot Camp podcast, I decided to "make lemonade" out of what I had been through. My therapist says, "We are as sick as our secrets." (Alcoholics Anonymous) I decided to set my story free with the hope that it could help just one person who may be experiencing mental health issues from Lyme.

Over the years, I've received so many messages from people asking for advice and sharing their stories with me that I decided to continue with my education and obtain a degree in Forensic Psychology so that I could study crisis intervention to help others recover from traumatic events and police interactions. I hope to start my own business in the future to help others who have been through similar experiences as I, especially Lyme patients. I also hope to share my story so

39: The Board of Pharmacy

that people can see the signs of and recognize what to look for before the illness reaches a crisis.

Other Thoughts

I have begun advocacy work through the virtual Lyme fly-in, held by the Center for Lyme Action and was able to listen to many stories during the training process. I took notes on the key things people stated that identified what is needed to make progress in the Lyme world.

The first request made was for accurate testing, especially for the initial movement into a late stage. Current testing only looks for acute Lyme and, as we know, is not accurate. A new test (from IGeneX) was just FDA approved and is called the IgG Immunoblot kit. This test has a sensitivity of 93%. In addition, a highly accurate Bartonella test has been released. This is an exciting step in the right direction.

The second request made was for more education for physicians. In medical school, most doctors receive minimal information about Lyme disease and tick-borne illnesses. Additional courses or certificates made available to educate doctors on how to identify, diagnose, and treat tick borne disease would help educate the medical system, preventing people from suffering undiagnosed for years.

The third request made was for affordable Lyme treatment. My treatment worked, but not every family has hundreds of thousands of dollars to spend on treatment. We need treatment that is effective and is affordable.

The fourth need that was recommended was for peer-reviewed studies for chronic late-stage Lyme. Most of the research and testing is focused on acute Lyme, and those of us in late-stage do not receive the attention or research we deserve. This is needed.

The fifth request was for tick surveillance. The CDC claimed there was no Lyme in California. The Bay Area Lyme Foundation did their own research to screen California from a lab located in Colorado. Infected ticks were found in California. In 2021, infected ticks were discovered on a beach in Los Angeles. There is Lyme in California, if one is willing to look for it.

One request from the experienced advocates was to establish a center for chronic disease institute at NIH. For a long time, as a Lyme patient, I was angry at these institutions for failing us. As advocates, we were instructed that our duty was to "make friends" with the politicians and the institutions. If we educate by calmly telling our stories to win people over, we can make change. That's exactly what the Center for Lyme Action is doing. From its creation in 2019, they have increased Lyme funding for Lyme and tick-borne disease from $59M in FY20 to $177.5M in FY24.

Many of the aids working for Congress, with whom we met, had no idea of the number of constituents in their own counties that suffer from Lyme disease. Congress had no idea how devastating the illness is. People in California have committed suicide resulting from their Lyme diagnosis, in addition to multiple instances of medical assistance with dying by choice. A medical bio bank exists that accepts tissue donations of those who have passed with Lyme disease, as well as tissue donations from post-op Lyme patients.

You can find information about this at the Bay Area Lyme Foundation. People suffer and turn to these devastating options because the system failed them. Now that I am healthy enough to help, I feel it is my responsibility to advocate and speak up for those who cannot. I also hope my story offers one of hope. I laid in bed for 3 years unable to walk and talk most days, hopeless and believing this was my fate.

39: The Board of Pharmacy

Medical breakthroughs are coming. Education of our politicians and government agencies, like the CDC and NIH, are coming.

Keep your hope intact and watch for the positive changes that are on the horizon for Lyme disease patient-warriors.

Dental Health and Lyme

My teeth were completely destroyed—I have IV doxycycline to thank for it. The enamel became cavernous with black and green holes. I had to go through most of rehab with my teeth looking like this. Help from the dentist was only temporary, as he would fill the holes, only for the teeth to turn black again.

Suddenly, my gums grew red and puffy. Multiple times, the dentists attempted to fix my teeth without results. After a visit with a parasite practitioner, the importance of seeing a biological dentist was suggested. I had never heard of this. As it turned out, the biological dentist was the first who knew what to do.

Biological dentists use nontoxic products that are made in the United States. The plan? Six veneers up top to fix my smile, as well as to lightly drill off all of the work the previous dentist had done—a treatment that caused the gum irritation.

It worked.

Gently bleaching the rest of my teeth, along with the work mentioned above, my smile was restored to its original state. Thankfully, this dentist was Lyme-literate and diagnoses people with Lyme and parasites by using a floss test.

Lyme can live in the gums. The floss test is called **DNA CONNEXIONS COMPREHENSIVE ORAL TEST** which tests for Lyme and coinfections in the gums. This dentist also introduced me to ozone treatment for chronically inflamed gums. I now go for cleanings every three months with ozone treatment that is directly applied to the gum line to keep the mouth healthy and germ free.

I highly recommend a biological dentist if you are dealing with mold, Lyme, parasites, or heavy metals.

Prevention

Prevention is the only way to completely protect oneself from developing late-stage chronic Lyme. Covering up appropriately when entering known tick-infested areas is crucial. Obligatory surveillance and accurately labeled infested areas should be mandatory. Clothing should be removed and thrown in the dryer after leaving a wooded or trail area. Perform thorough tick checks after hikes and in areas where you are at risk of a tick bite.

Should you find an attached tick, I recommend Tick Boot Camp's Tick Bite Blueprint that explains clearly everything you need to know about avoiding ticks and treating tick bites.

Always remove ticks with tweezers and pull out with steady even pressure. This prevents any pieces from being left behind inside the skin. Always send the tick off to a lab for testing (not medical advice but expert advice based on personal experience). If I were to get bitten again, I would do a round of oral antibiotics—symptomatic or not. Doing so prevents the disease from progressing. Involve a Lyme-literate doctor from the start.

The faster you can jump on treatment, the better the chances you have of preventing chronic late-stage Lyme. I would not wait for a bull's-eye rash. Even the CDC admits that not everyone with Lyme develops this symptom.

A relatively new herbal product that is recommended by an LLMD called, "As soon as you are bit" (ASAB). It can be found at https://shop.turnpaughhwc.com/products/asab. This

39: The Board of Pharmacy

is an herbal treatment used to prevent Lyme and associated co-infections.

Another option is Samsura Tick Immune support for an acute tick bite, which prevents all illnesses from invading the body. These are herbal options for those who are hesitant to go with antibiotics. Stevia leaf extract is also an effective antimicrobial agent against Borrelia Burgdorferi.

The TiCK MiTT is a new invention by a Lyme Warrior to help remove ticks from your body and pets after a walk in a possible tick-infested area. It can be found at tickmitt.com. Center for Lyme advocate and Lyme warrior, Meghan Bradshaw, shares her list for gardening and outdoor activities: pants tucked into her insect shield socks, light colored long sleeve shirt and hat, permethrin-treated boots, spraying herself down with 3 Moms Organics Tick and Insect Repellant from head to toe, and treating her yard with Tick Warriors Eco-Friendly Pest Protection.

Lyme and families

Lyme disease and tick-borne illnesses are often seen within family members. Lyme can be passed from mother to baby. Family members vacation or live in a common location where they are often exposed to ticks. Some people believe Lyme can be sexually transmitted, particularly after a study released that showed a small number of couples, both having the same strains of Lyme disease. This could also be due to couples that were exposed to ticks in the same area. More research needs to be done. My doctor doesn't believe this is likely and if it is, he believes it is extremely rare. If you are actively infected, it doesn't hurt to be safe and protect your partner until more is learned about this. Read more: https://pubmed.ncbi.nlm.nih.gov/28690828/

If you have a family member with Lyme or tick-borne disease and are symptomatic, get tested and immediately seek out a Lyme-literate doctor (LLMD).

While writing this book, multiple people close to me have been diagnosed with tick-borne illness. One associate also tested positive for black mold and mold illness. One person found the tick and broke out with the classic bull's-eye rash. The other individual never recalled ever receiving a tick bite.

The CDC recommends 10-14 days of antibiotics to prevent Lyme from progressing. In the Lyme community, this is not considered sufficient treatment. A longer antibiotic protocol that runs for four to six weeks is usually recommended in Lyme circles. I asked my LLMD about this, who stated that 21 days minimum to receive antibiotic therapy is highly recommended after any tick bite to prevent chronic Lyme.

Morgellons

Morgellons is largely dismissed in the medical community as "delusional parasitosis." I had never heard of Morgellons until I began searching for answers. This occurred after lesions developed all over my body.

Morgellons The Legitimization of a Disease by Dr. Ginger Savely is a book that provided answers. At the time I was diagnosed, Morgellons was barely discussed and the symptoms often dismissed as psychological. This was true for me as my chief complaint was lesions when I checked into the ER. The doctors dismissed my complaints and handed my dad a list of psychiatrists. The medical professionals in the ER believed that I had been cutting holes in my skin and intentionally inserting things that looked like fibers beneath the skin. Their premise was mental illness.

39: The Board of Pharmacy

Nowadays, NIH studies have proven the link between Lyme and Morgellons.

Lyme Mexico on YouTube offers insight into the illness, discussing symptoms and causes openly, breaking the stigma that exists. The only treatment for the lesions I experienced was to treat the root cause: Lyme disease.

I tried many lotions and potions, and nothing seemed to help until I received stem cells. Miraculously, while in the hospital, my skin began to heal.

Sadly, Morgellons also causes confusion, and sometimes induces delusions or mental health issues, severe pain under the skin, and a crawling sensation under the skin. Understanding the complexity of Lyme disease and Morgellons is crucial to combating the debilitating symptomatology and the illnesses that result from a tick bite.

The Trauma of the Holocaust Victim

Holocaust survivors pass down their trauma.

A goal of mine is to break generational trauma. It happens in all families in one way or another. I think to break the narrative that we cannot discuss personal problems is a great way to start. Silence and turning a blind eye to the devastation that occurs with traumatic events is akin to agreeing with it. We must collectively be the voice for those who cannot speak for themselves.

Lyme literate therapist Christina Kantzavelos discusses the quote by Dr. Gabor Mate that states, "Children aren't traumatized because they're hurt—they're traumatized because they're alone with their pain." She continues to bring up the point that trauma is less likely to be stored in the body if children have one trusted person with whom to talk their problems through.

Kaitlyn Oleinik

I come from a family of Missouri farmers with English, German, and Irish roots on one side and Ashkenazi Jewish Holocaust survivors on the other. My grandfather was a resistance leader during the Holocaust in Poland and took refuge hiding in the woods to escape the concentration camps.

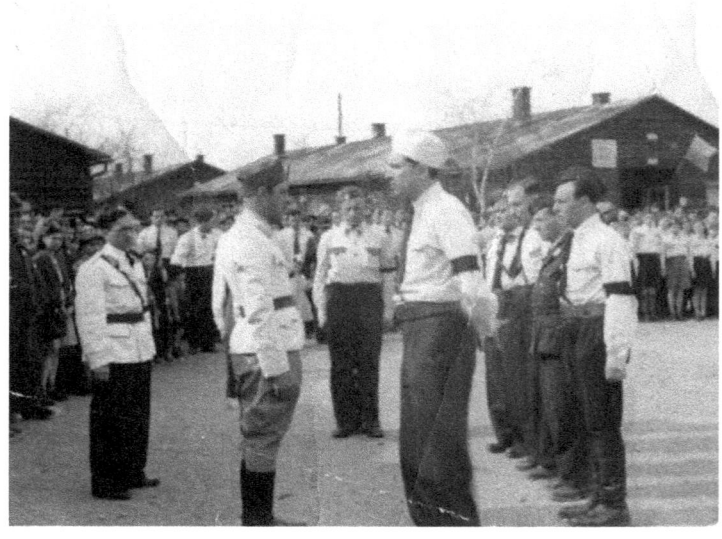

Grandpa Zelik (front left in tall boots) in Displaced Persons Camp he helped run in Linz, Austria

The Olejník-Bobrov Brigade went out to avenge their loved ones killed by the Nazis. My grandfather lost his first family to a Nazi firing squad (we learned this later through my Great Uncle Norman). This took place long before he met my grandmother, which took place during the Holocaust. Eventually, they had children—my father and uncle while living in a Displaced Persons camp in Austria. Both my grandfather and grandmother rarely discussed their experiences, even keeping their tragic past from their own children.

39: The Board of Pharmacy

Studies show:

The extreme trauma that survivors of the Holocaust faced, and face have impacts on their children and grandchildren: Emotionally, through PTSD symptoms and mental disorders; and physically, through stress modifiers in their genes. Hopefully more research will be done, so that we can better understand how the Holocaust affected our understanding of trauma and the generational implications of it (Hoyer & Searce, 2024).

Trauma is passed down through epigenetics. My great uncle Norman allowed me to record his version of surviving the war and my great aunt Blanche offered her testimony to USC's Shoah documentary, which I have saved. To bear testimony is a great act, if one is comfortable doing so.

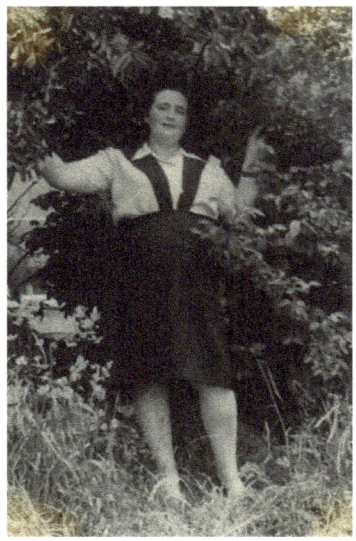 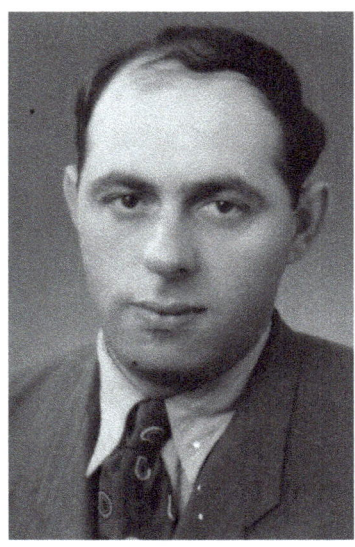

Grandma Bertha & Grandpa Zelik (Holocaust Survivors)

In 2023, I happened to be in Israel on October 7th and faced my own war experience. I was scared at what being in a war zone would do to my mental health but made it through the two weeks. Soon, I made my way to Greece and eventually back home.

I was diagnosed with an acute stress response and used therapy as a tool to prevent the further diagnosis of post-traumatic stress disorder (PTSD). What has happened on both sides, since that day, breaks my heart. People deserve to live in a peaceful place with shelter and safety.

I think going to therapy and working through generational trauma, even having a trusted ally to talk with, is crucial for initiating the healing process and the outcome of healed families.

Clear signs exist giving evidence that trauma from one generation can be passed down to future generations in families. Studies conducted at New York's Mount Sinai Hospital (led by Rachel Yehuda) considered the possibility of genetically passing on trauma experienced through torture suffered at Nazi concentration camps and/or through hiding during WWII (Thomson, 2015). Genetic tests that looked at these survivor's children show gene changes that this research identified as "only attributed to Holocaust exposure in the parents."

The idea that traumatic experience is passed through generations is daunting. Perhaps modern-day post-traumatic stress disorder (PTSD) and depressive or panic attack symptoms common to individuals living today can be attributed in part to their predecessors' distressing lives. These genetic contributions need further research to identify which gene and how the trauma is processed in families. Doing so will likely enable

39: The Board of Pharmacy

medical and psychiatric professionals to treat those who suffer from distress that originates in someone else's trauma.

Just a thought…

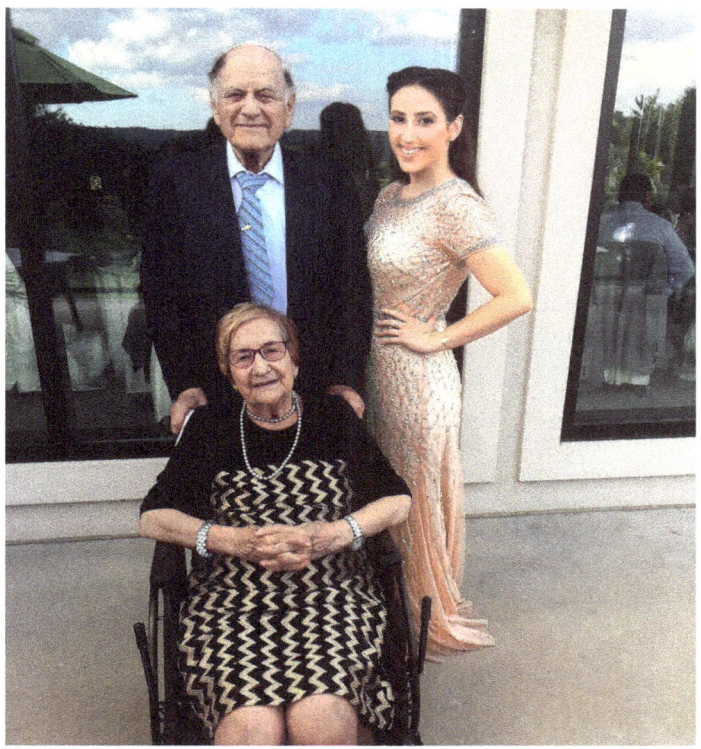

Great Uncle Norm & Great Aunt Blanche
(Holocaust survivors), and Me

End Statement

A change in research needs to shift to focus on patients who already have reached a late-stage, tried typical treatments, and are failing to get better.

Do NOT give up hope!

Kaitlyn

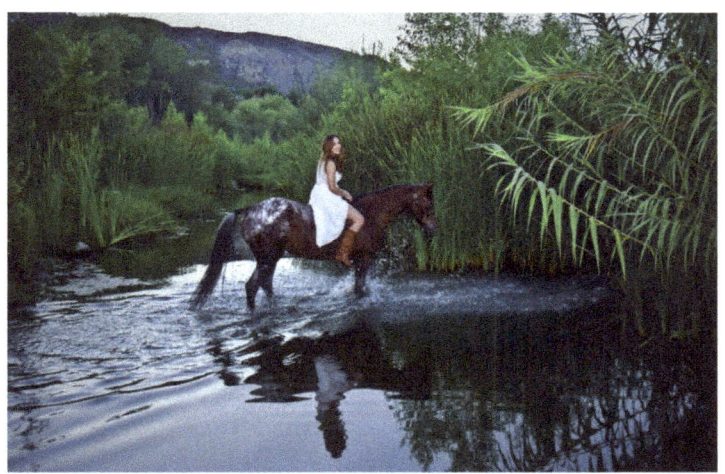

Photo credit Lia Ann Segerblom

*please note: These comments are given as an informational resource only. I do not promote specific treatments.

Kaitlyn Oleinik

MEDICAL ADVICE DISCLAIMER

DISCLAIMER: THIS BOOK DOES NOT PROVIDE MEDICAL ADVICE. I am not a doctor or medical professional. The information, including but not limited to, text, graphics, images and other material contained in this book are solely of the opinion of the author and for informational purposes only. No material contained herein is intended to be a substitute for professional medical advice, diagnosis or treatment. ALWAYS SEEK THE ADVICE OF YOUR PHYSICIAN or other qualified health care provider with any questions you may have regarding a medical condition or treatment, and before undertaking a new health care regimen, and never disregard professional medical advice or delay seeking it because of something you have read on the pages in this book.

References

American Psychological Association. (2022, June 1). Unraveling the mystery of Lyme disease. *Monitor on Psychology*, *53*(4). https://www.apa.org/monitor/2022/06/feature-lyme-disease

Anger & Lyme disease: What to know about Lyme rage (2017, March 2). Global Lyme Alliance. https://www.globallymealliance.org/blog/its-ok-to-be-angry-lyme-disease

Carrasco, J. P., & Aguilar, E. J. (2024). Antibiomania: A case report of a manic episode potentially induced by the interaction of clarithromycin and amoxicillin during H. Pylori eradication therapy. *Actas espanolas de psiquiatria*, *52*(1), 57–59.

Cefaclor (n.d.) RxList. https://www.rxlist.com/cefaclor/generic-drug.htm

Center for Disease Control (2024, May 14). About parvovirus B19. *CDC Parvovirus B19 and Fifth Disease*. https://www.cdc.gov/parvovirus-b19/about/index.html

Clarizio, G. (2016, March 19). *Mystery diagnosis Lyme disease part 1* [video file]. YouTube. https://youtu.be/I8UR_iLEaZ4?feature=shared

Cleveland Clinic (2022, September 9). *Postural orthostatic tachycardia syndrome (POTS)*. https://my.clevelandclinic.org/health/diseases/16560-postural-orthostatic-tachycardia-syndrome-pots

Grier, T. (2019, March 28). Investigating connections between Lyme disease and dementia. *Lyme Disease. https://www.lymedisease.org/lyme-disease-dementia-grier/*

Griffin, L. (2011, May 15). Today's virtual walk to raise awareness for Lyme disease. *Patch*. https://patch.com/new-jersey/millburn/virtual-walk-to-raise-awareness-for-lyme-disease

Hoyer, J. & Searce, T. (2024, June 14). The holocaust and generational trauma. *University of Arkansas*. https://howdidtheholocaustaffect.uark.edu/2024/06/14/the-holocaust-and-generational-trauma/#:~:text=Overall%2C%20studies%20show%20that%20the,stress%20modifiers%20in%20their%20genes

Karatzias, T., Shevlin, M., Hyland, P., Brewin, C.R., Cloitre, M., Bradley, A., Kitchiner, N.J., Jumbe, S., Bisson, J. I., & Roberts, N.P. (2018), The role of negative cognitions, emotion regulation strategies, and attachment style in complex post-traumatic stress disorder: Implications for new and existing therapies. Br J Clin Psychol, 57: 177-185. https://doi.org/10.1111/bjc.12172

Kerstholt, M., Vrijmoeth, H., Lachmandas, E., Oosting, M., Lupse, M., Flonta, M., Dinarello, C. A., Netea, M. G., & Joosten, L. A. B. (2018). Role of glutathione metabolism in host defense against *Borrelia burgdorferi* infection. *Proceedings of the National Academy of Sciences of the United States of America*, *115*(10). https://doi.org/10.1073/pnas.1720833115

Kinderlehrer, D. (2024, September 24). Lyme disease and mental illness, Infections causing eating disorders. *Project Lyme*. https://projectlyme.org/lyme-and-mental-illness-infections-causing-eating-disorders/

Kostolansky S, Waymack JR. Erythema Infectiosum. (2023, July 31). StatPearls [Internet]. *StatPearls Publishing*. https://www.ncbi.nlm.nih.gov/books/NBK513309/

Macri, A. & Crane, J. S. (2023, June 28). Parvoviruses. *StatPearls*. https://www.ncbi.nlm.nih.gov/books/NBK482245/

Mardhiyah, A., Philip, K., Mediani, H. S., & Yosep, I. (2020). The association between hope and quality of life among adolescents with chronic diseases: A systematic review. *Child health nursing research*, *26*(3), 323–328. https://doi.org/10.4094/chnr.2020.26.3.323

Melville, M. (2025, January 15). Article on Hope and Wellness (provided for *The Chicago School of Professional Psychology*). https://martirnadvisor.com/

Middelveen, M. J., Bandoski, C., Burke, J., Sapi, E., Filush, K. R., Wang, Y., Franco, A., Mayne, P. J., & Stricker, R. B. (2015). Exploring the association between Morgellons disease and Lyme disease: identification of Borrelia burgdorferi in Morgellons disease patients. *BMC dermatology*, *15*(1), 1. https://doi.org/10.1186/s12895-015-0023-0

Peak, T. (2024, June 10). Bartonella DNA found in blood of patients with psychosis. *North Carolina State University*. https://www.sciencedaily.com/releases/2024/06/240610140158.htm.

Radolf, J. D., Strle, K., Lemieux, J. E., & Strle, F. (2021). Lyme disease in humans. *Current Issues in Molecular Biology* 42(1). https://doi.org/10.21775/cimb.042.333

Shor, S., Green, C., Szantyr, B., Phillips, S., Liegner, K., Burrascano, J. J., Jr, Bransfield, R., & Maloney, E. L. (2019). Chronic Lyme disease: An evidence-based definition by the ILADS working group. *Antibiotics (Basel, Switzerland)*, *8*(4), 269. https://doi.org/10.3390/antibiotics8040269

Sweet, P. L. (2019). The sociology of gaslighting. *Americal Sociological Review* 84(5). https://www.asanet.org/wp-content/uploads/attach/journals/oct19asrfeature.pdf

Talkington, J., & Nickell, S. P. (1999). Borrelia burgdorferi spirochetes induce mast cell activation and cytokine release. *Infection and immunity*, *67*(3), 1107–1115. https://doi.org/10.1128/IAI.67.3.1107-1115.1999

Thomson, H. (2015, August 21). Study of Holocaust survivors finds trauma passed on to children's genes. *The Guardian*. https://www.theguardian.com/science/2015/aug/21/study-of-holocaust-survivors-finds-trauma-passed-on-to-childrens-genes

Tsafir, J. S. (2017, August 3). Mold toxicity: A common cause of psychiatric symptoms. *Psychology Today*. https://www.psychologytoday.com/us/blog/holistic-psychiatry/201708/mold-toxicity-a-common-cause-of-psychiatric-symptoms

About the Author

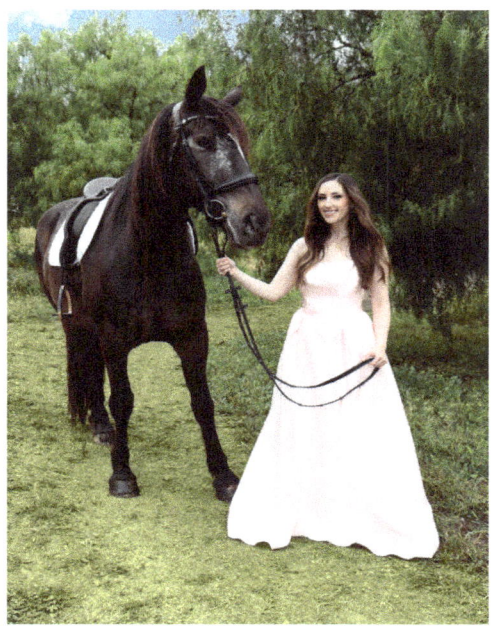

Kaitlyn Oleinik, known to many as *GoldenKait*, survived Lyme disease and now advocates for other survivors. With a voice shaped by resilience, and a perspective rooted in empathy, Kaitlyn brings a unique lens to her creative and academic work. Her journey through chronic illness has not only shaped her identity but also deepened her mission to amplify underrepresented voices and challenge the current system to support Lyme Disease patients.

Kaitlyn Oleinik

Kaitlyn's hobbies include equestrian events, singing, and songwriting. She is currently pursuing her Master of Science Degree in Forensic Psychology.

Revival: My Journey with Neuropsychiatric Lyme Disease is her debut book, and it reflects the complexity, heart, and strength she carries into every project. It is Kaitlyn's hope for change and the understanding of the journey that is late-stage neuropsychiatric Lyme disease.

Follow me on Instagram: @GoldenKait

www.ingramcontent.com/pod-product-compliance
Lightning Source LLC
Chambersburg PA
CBHW052029030426
42337CB00027B/4921